LIVING
HELL

LIVING
HELL

The Truth about AIDS and HIV

JOSEFINA GUARDIA

iUniverse, Inc.
Bloomington

Living Hell
The Truth about AIDS and HIV

iUniverse books may be ordered through booksellers or by contacting:

iUniverse
1663 Liberty Drive
Bloomington, IN 47403
www.iuniverse.com
1-800-Authors (1-800-288-4677)

ISBN: 978-1-4502-8855-2 (sc)
ISBN: 978-1-4502-8857-6 (dj)
ISBN: 978-1-4502-8856-9 (ebk)

Printed in the United States of America

iUniverse rev. date: 02/23/2011

1. How this book came to be

Hello, my name is Josefina. For quite some time now, I have been soul searching and contemplating about my life. This book was written from the heart and is presented with Spiritual Love. Let me tell you a little about myself and how the desire to write "LIVING HELL ... AIDS (H.I.V.)" came about ...

I was born in 1954 in Barcelona, Spain, where I lived for the first 18 years of my life. My brother, two sisters and are blessed with wonderful, loving parents. At the time, our neighborhood was a nice place to grow up. As it stands today, I have two handsome sons and a precious daughter. We are all simple people ... we're Christians!

Professionally, I am a Nurses Assistant. On weekends, I work part-time as a security guard. My personality is and always has been that of a generous and caring orderly person. I love plants, and enjoy knitting, cooking and listening to Christian Music. I also enjoy helping others and giving!

EVER SINCE I HAVE BECOME A NURSE ASSISTANT, and I have been one for three years now, I have felt that the patients needed something more than a doctor. They needed for someone to really listen to them, to demonstrate their concern and caring for them. In the short period of time that I have been working in the hospital, I have seen many people die. What really breaks my heart is seeing the surviving family members. Alright, many have seen these things happen. But many may not have seen, or paid attention to, when patients are by themselves ... ALL ALONE!

However, what I really at this time want to tell you about is the H.I.V. virus, also known as AIDS. The truth is of course, that no one wants to have this dreaded illness. But, the problem is how to live with AIDS.

I have a terrible aching pain inside for these patients that do have AIDS. They are so alone! People seem to treat them worse than lepers of ancient times. But there is no reason to treat them this way.

You see, there are only a few ways of contracting the H.I.V. virus and it's nothing like that of leprosy or any other highly contagious disease. With the AIDS virus, a person can get it through sharing needles (in the case of intravenous drug users), direct blood (and body fluids) contact with an AIDS infected person with cuts, scratches, or through other direct avenues to the blood system of non-AIDS infected individuals. Also, constant sexual activity with many different partners enhances ones chances of acquiring the AIDS virus.

In hospital situations, it has been seen that someone stuck by a needle that was used on an AIDS infected patient contracting the H.I.V. virus. However, it has also been proven, that many people believe that by giving a hug or a kiss to someone infected with AIDS, that they too will get the virus. . Once again, this sickness is not like leprosy of the Middle Ages. I beg everyone to please open your eyes to the facts of this virus that has everyone afraid to come in contact with AIDS victims.

There are so many people that have it and that are getting closer to death with each second that ticks on the clock. Their friends and families abandon them to die a very frightening, extremely painful and lonesome death. This is terrible and heartbreaking to know that their family members and very close friends forsake them due to ignorance.

I work with these "infected" persons nearly everyday and it is painful to see how they suffer alone, not having anyone who will give them a hug and tell them not to worry ... and I love you! I personally, am going to help them in all the ways that is possible for me to keep up moral to help them get the most out of what little life time that they may still have remaining. Sometimes I'll bring them some candy, pastries or a homemade gift that I have made for that individual. And they truly enjoy it, and thank me!

Together we share the moments of joy and happiness and ... the moments of pain.

AIDS is an illness that is horrible and very painful. At times short, at other times it is prolonged. It all depends on where it attacks first. I suffer when seeing them tormented in this manner; it's a death that is truly cruel, drawing one's compassion for them and how they ache. I try my best to console them – night after night, with these fevers so high, with the vomiting and begging God to have mercy on them. Some have asked me to teach them to pray; others cry in my arms. Others ask that I give them a hug and want to hear me tell them that there is someone who loves and cares about them.

It's painful, for most do have family. I'm the one that is together with them in their last moments of life holding their hand and speaking to them and calming their fears of death as they die. Part of me dies right along with them. This is what motivates me to write this book. I ask Almighty God to guide me as I write that these words will touch the hearts of some people that have family or friends with AIDS. It's not necessary for you to abandon your very close loved ones in the hospitals simply because they have the AIDS virus!

We also have prisoners that have H.I.V. and with the collaboration and blessings from all of them, I will write this book. My hope is that these testimonies about them can help you. I have asked patients, and received their permission from them, to present their testimonies and how they feel about being condemned to death with the AIDS virus. I have a few of them that are my favorites. It's like children in a way, how there are always a few that seem to get closer to you than the others. However, I do love them all, especially for their courage and faith!

I would like with time to be able to open a place where they would be cared for, if it be God's will. With His blessings, this place could be a place where they could feel happy and could enjoy their final days in peace. Where they would be able to search for spiritual peace, as well as be physically comfortable. For them, the road is short, very short, and very painful. Only God knows how much we suffer together. I'm always close to them, and I understand that it's not easy for them to live this kind of life. I always think that whatever I do for them now, will be brought with them into the hereafter.

I pray daily to Our Heavenly Father that people will have compassion toward all AIDS victims, because they truly suffer tremendously. It is as though they are being tormented in Hell's Fire daily.

Some of the people who have given me their testimony and permission to use it in this book may have already left to be with the Lord. Others are nearing that point, and still some are only beginning their trip through the Valley of the Shadow of Death!

Dear God, please help me to get out the message of Your Saving Grace through Your Son Jesus Christ, and be with these that are begging for your mercy. Grant them oh Lord, your Grace as their time nears.

Amen.

2. Uncharted territory

BEING COMPLETELY HONEST WITH YOU right from the beginning, I must admit that I have no knowledge or experience as a writer; however I do have something to pass on to you. I will do this as if we were sitting down together exchanging experiences over coffee. Going directly to the point, the things I want to talk about are of people having AIDS that have trouble telling their loved ones that they have contracted the illness or refuse to tell them at all. The book's main purpose is for us all to have a greater understanding and learn the facts about AIDS in order that we may feel free to express our compassion for those affected and their families.

I believe that people with AIDS should share that information with their families and not worry about somehow passing the illness on to them. Then they would be allowing themselves and their family members to openly express their love and support without fear. We MUST all understand that if care is taken no one else will contract the virus. God only knows that I have no idea on how to write a book, and especially one on this subject, being only a nurse's assistant. But I am the one that is constantly working intimately with them on a daily basis, sharing their happy and sad painful moments and being by their sides during long hours and nights.

They are like children when they are sick, calling for mommy. This is how I feel. Their families, don't have any idea of how they spend their nights. But I know, because I am there. The pain is so strong that they cannot withstand it. If only they could see them, they would probably understand what I'm talking about. I feel like an adopted mother to them, and I thank God for it, because the pain is released.

For the most part, a lot of them don't want to tell their families, or they don't know how to say it. Sometimes, some tell their families, only to be abandoned by their families like dogs. I think it is because they are scared and they don't know the facts of this sickness. But, if they knew all the facts, then they would understand that there is no need to worry; there are only a few ways to get infected by it. Only their ignorance causes them to stay away. They don't know any better.

But, I hope because I took my time to write this book, maybe they will understand this sickness . Maybe they will help their loved ones and stop abandoning them. Perhaps they will learn, and begin to understand and care for their family members with love and patience.

I don't know what to say to you, my friends, other than that we need to help those that are in need. I feel very bad because I cannot do it alone, and there are many that are dying every day. I ask God to help me. What I want to tell you is that we need to get together and do it together. Maybe one day one of them will be be our son or daughter. Can you see why I'm telling you this? Only God knows what is going to happen.

We should pay more attention to our children. I know it's very hard to understand them, but if we don't try we will never know. We can help them by telling them what is going on in this world. I have a 16-year-old son, a 14–year-old daughter. And I am really worried about them because this world is not safe for them. We have to protect our children from this sickness.

A lot of times when I'm working and one of my patients calls me I go and talk with him and he tells me how he feels about this sickness and he asks me a lot of questions and I don't know what to tell him. Because I know he is going to die, I try to comfort him as much as I can. It's very hard. So he asks me if I can give him a hug and a kiss and I do it. The he cries like a little boy and thanks me for loving and caring for him. He looks me in the eyes and says "Thank you. God Bless you for bringing happiness into my life!" Then he goes back to sleep knowing somebody loves him. When I go back to my seat, I have a lot of time to think. I end up feeling very bad because I'm taking somebody else's place – because I am taking a mother's place.

And that's not my place.

What I want to say is, don't be embarrassed to have sons or daughters with HIV. The truth is, this is a horrible disease that requires love and understanding. We should help those with HIV as much as possible. For example, I always attempted to teach my children when they see people injecting drugs and I explain to them what happens to. I even take my children to where I work so they can see for themselves what happens to people with AIDS – but I have done so with love and care so they understand that I show them this for their own good.

So that there are no misunderstandings, I tell them if someone molests them that they should tell me. That it is nothing to be ashamed of, rather, it is better to prevent something than need to cure it.

In many cases of molested or violated children, I have discovered that when they are young, they develop a bad attitude from other children that only worsens as they get older. Many of them turn to drugs to forget what happened to them. This leads to their own self-destruction simply because they could not tell anyone that they had a thorn in their heart - for who would believe a child? So, many parents do not know about the abuse, and as the children grow older some become homosexuals and others turn to drugs to forget that shadow that follows them. They wish to change the world, but unfortunately they don't realize that they cannot change what happened to them. I would like to help all of those who are in need of affection and be able to tell them that I understand how they feel.

I know what it is like to carry that shadow, for I too have been there, but thank God it passed and I did not need drugs or other things to get out of that shadow.

We cannot think even for a moment that they wish to live in that manner. AIDS is not a sin, it is a disease. As Jesus said in the Bible "he who had not committed any sin cast the first stone." We cannot condemn anyone. We cannot condemn them because we are all human and we have all made mistakes.

Unfortunately, none of us are perfect. What I wish to say with this book is: open your hearts and allow these poor unfortunates enter. Give them affection and understanding. Take care of them because they need you. I alone cannot do it all.

All of the accounts that I have written in this book are real. All of them need someone that gives them encouragement to keep going; it is evil's goal to keep them coming back to the street corner.

Sometimes I think no matter what situation I am in, I cannot change the world but God gives me the strength and energy to keep going. That helps me. Many times I feel depressed and have said, *To hell with everything,* because I cannot do this anymore because no one knows what it feels inside when I think of all those people who have died in my arms.

When I return home in the morning, I go directly to my children's bedrooms to give them a kiss and try to lessen what occurred. They know someone died that night and tell me that they love me and that I am the most beautiful mother in the entire world. They kiss and hug me. They say and do all of these things because they see the pain written on my face. But my mind is not present. My heart races like a locomotive thinking about the patients who are dying and I can not do anything for them.

Many have caused me to reach my breaking point. I have cried inconsolably and I have considered not returning to work, as I could no longer bear watching them suffer in such a cruel and horrible way. In truth, no one knows how I suffered for them, but then I realize I cannot abandon them as now is when they need me most. I pray so that God would give me strength to keep going.

I was exhausted physically and morally; but then it occurred to me there was something I could probably do for them. If I could open a center, perhaps volunteers could provide them with assistance.

I asked God to guide my hand as I do not wish to write anything that would offend anyone. I only wish to say the truth. All of the testimonies I have written in this book were possible with the help of many volunteers with AIDS who desire to help young people so they do not commit the same mistakes. I give them thanks because, in truth, what we want is that they do not remain in the dark rather that they see the truth given they are our future and if we do not teach them what is happening in the world they cannot remove the blinders from over their eyes.

I remember when I was in Spain, especially when I was in a bad location. In Barcelona, there is a place called Las Ramblas – the Boulevard. During the day it is a marvelous place – like a long trip where no cars go by and it has the largest stores, with flowers of many colors; all kinds of animals of every color one can imagine. There are ice cream parlors and people selling imitation jewelry and people reading the newspaper seated on the benches. Artists are painting beautiful things in the streets. Well, you cannot imagine such beautiful and rare things you can find there. But, when it starts to get dark, everyone picks up their things and quickly disappear as if the wind had carried them off. And now, a new life begins.

Everything that was once beautiful is now horrifying. Bars open and the streets fill with all kinds of strange people, some without scruples – people who would murder for a dollar. There are people who sell themselves to buy the drugs that have them enslaved. It is not only the women who sell themselves, but also men. I lived on one of those streets for a while and we could not go out at night because of shootings; there was also drug use, even in the middle of the street.

I have seen in Spain and America how drugs eat at drug addicts little by little. What I wish to tell you is that drugs are everywhere – and so is AIDS. All we can do is pray so that someday someone discovers a cure for this illness that is ending our beloved's lives; those beings who mothers carried in their wombs for nine months.

Who knows; someday we can find ourselves in the same situation they are in. I give everything, for we are all to love one another and that is a mandate that is written. *"Love your neighbor as you love yourself,"* I love them all very much - no one knows the pain and suffering they carry in their hearts.

3. Israel's story

Tonight is a night like any other and I am speaking with a new patient. He wants to tell me how he got AIDS. He is the son of country folk, honest and hard working. His parents had three children and they wished to educate all three the best way possible. They were poor and had no money, but it isn't necessary to have money to be honest and good. They grew up as many of our children have, without an education and without work.

Israel, unlike his siblings, has some issues. He kept bad company and when one keeps bad company, one ends up bad. He intended to lead a righteous life like many others, but in this life everything is very difficult. When he became an adult, he found a girlfriend. Like most couples, after a couple of years, they decided to get married. They did not have the good fortune of being one of a thousand; being poor. But, they loved each other and that was most important to them.

In time, they had a daughter and it seemed everything was looking better. But the situation was getting worse. His wife abandoned him for another man. Israel was very confused and could not believe what was happening. He wanted to forget about his wife, but he needed someone to talk to in order to get over his loss. Eventually, without anyone to talk to, he found himself facing something he didn't wish to face He found himself face-to-face with a monster known as drugs.

Once he started using, he could not stop. Days of using soon turned into years. Every day he sank deeper into the mud. He had no power to do anything, as he had no good friends. He forgot about his daughter and what was left of his family. He forgot about himself. The only thing he could think about was the woman who destroyed his life. In reality, the only thing important to him was his drug habit. Each day he needed more and more. When he finally realized it, he was completely addicted and the years passed by.

There is a saying that says he who chooses badly ends badly. He would tell me *"I feel like a sardine in a can and I am paying for everything I have done. Everything started with a small problem and now for me there aren't many experiences left. I have HIV and nobody wants me. There isn't much time for me; my day grows nearer. When I leave I wish to go with my daughter and her husband as I wish to live my final days of my life with them. I know very well that when people find out I have HIV they will suffer and I cannot forgive myself for that. But with God's help I will come out ahead and now I am not alone as I have found peace I have been looking for. I know that God is by my side and with his help I can begin a new life."*

4. Things are so similar, yet so different.

Apart from all these patients whom I appreciate so much, there are others who I only spoke with four or five times. All of them begin on the same path and end up the same way. Each one of them have a different life and a different history.

There are some who know how to change, but there are others who have no memory. We had a patient with a tumor on his palate. He was HIV positive and often when he put something in his mouth, he bled so much I became frightened. He was like that for a month. After what seemed like a thousand x-rays, the doctors decided to give him chemotherapy. It was horrible. The poor man suffered a great deal. It was a daily torture with a great deal of medicine, yet his illness progressed as if they gave him nothing at all. I don't know how he could endure it, yet he remained in that critical state for a long time. He began to respond to treatment and they returned him to prison. Each case is different, some die quickly; others live five months.

Another day, another new patient was gravely ill, in reality he was dying. He wanted to have a sex change operation and was already injecting hormones. He wanted to become a woman. I don't think he was able to complete it as he was gravely ill, but the AIDS was alive and it was eating him alive little by little. Above all else, in this situation that he is in, I do not believe that he will last long. What I will never understand is how a man can get it in his head he wants to become a woman and be operated on? I am sure that this is not something of God. This, better said, is a grand abomination and while it gave me such pity, I do not think he knows God. That is the reason people do the oddest things. However, I do not know what could change a man's mind in this state. I normally had many conversations with him and he treated me with much respect always. He behaved very well with me, but to this present day I still don't understand why he wanted to become a woman.

Each day passes by and he continues to grow worse; I don't think he will last much longer. There are things in this life that we don't understand and others that we have begun to understand. Perhaps when he was young, someone abused him and that could be the cause of his confusion and he thought he was at fault that is why he decided to change his gender. Normally when a child is sexually abused, the child thinks he or she is at fault. That must be what affected him all of his life and since he did not become brave enough to tell anyone, he grew up with that problem in his mind and that the best thing for him would be a sex change operation.

Although I do not believe that is the best, (but who am I to judge anyone?) sometimes we do not know the reason why people do things of this kind. Neither do we know who their lives were no do we know how they were raised. There are too many things to consider and we should take into account. Sometimes it is easier to criticize a person than to help him.

It is sad, but it is reality. It seems people have become cold without interest in helping others. I believe that we should know about people before criticizing them. After all, none of know how we will end up.

A few days after I finished writing this part, he died. I felt very bad. He was very young and he had a full life ahead of him. Now he doesn't have any more worries as it is all over.

I don't know what will become of our children with so much modernization. They are all headed for hell and I do not know what is happening with our youth today – men want to become women and women want to become men. I don't know where we will end up. I think the world is coming to an end – self-destruction. It is incredible that little by little as time goes by things are going from bad to worse. There are more illnesses and more misery. I do not know where we will go to end it. It seems like a bad dream or movie but we need to wake up. This is reality! It is not a dream. I ask God for other paths, although people would ultimately do what they want.

In the world that we live in, everything appears rose colored and perfect, but unfortunately, it is not that way. So many things to worry about: work, raising children, the house, school and above all else the streets. The streets are the most important because those where our children learn what they should not. For them, everything is a game. But how wrong they are for in the streets they only learn the things they should not. The streets only bring many headaches for the parents.

The other day, I spoke with the two prisoners we have at the hospital over this very subject. One of them told me that he was born in the ghetto and that he has seen girls 12- and 13-year-old selling themselves for drugs. It is such a shame; they are in the beginning of life and already lost.

My God, what will we do? The truth is society does not give us much to choose from; we need to work constantly and we have very little time for our children. It is difficult for us to watch them constantly. I think it is quite arduous to see our children in this manner. Girls as young as 10 or 12-years-old are selling themselves in the street for a bag of drugs and others for food for their babies, for many of them are 12- years-old and have children of their own. They are babies raising babies and they continue using drugs.

I ask myself what the future will be for our children. I sincerely think there is no future for anyone for we do not even know when we will die.

5. Edgar's story

Edgar was one of my first patients. With all of my love, I dedicate this part of my book to him although he is no longer with us. His spirit lives on and will always be with us; as a patient, as a friend – as a brother in Christ.

When I began to work at the hospital, he was my first patient. Edgar was Puerto Rican. A pleasant man but with a nasty temper – although it is understandable, he had his reasons to be angry. Edgar spoke barely any English, so I was his interpreter. One day, he was so sick he called me to his bedside. I found him crying like a small child.

I asked him, *"What is wrong, why are you crying?"*

He replied, *"You know how to pray?"*

I said, *"Yes, of course."*

He then said, *"I want you to teach me how to pray."*

I told him I would, *"I am a Christian"*.

I asked him if he believed in Jesus Christ and he answered yes. So, I taught him how to pray. After an hour of prayer I asked him how he felt. He answered much better. He said, *"Thanks be to God, I feel a bit better,"* then immediately he began to sweat profusely. He began to have tremors of fear and broke into a crying spell like a small child.

He asked me to let him die. I felt as if my heart broke into a thousand pieces. I said I cannot do that. God is the only one that can truly help you. He looked at me with sadness in his eyes. Then he asked me when I pray and you ask God for something in particular, he would respond to you. I remained silent for a long time for I knew what he was going to ask me. I looked into his eyes and I told him, *"Normally if everything depended on what I asked for …"* but before I could finish, he begged me to ask God to have mercy on him and to take him back to heaven soon.

By now, he had no more strength to carry on. With each moment that passed he grew weaker. He repeated constantly that he could not go on anymore – that he was tired of so much suffering. I told him I could not ask God for that. He looked at my face and responded that I was very kind to him. We spoke for hours about his family because they did not know he had AIDS. I told him not to worry because no one would tell them if he didn't want them to, but his family was always on his mind – especially his mother. The next day, I met his mother and I became close to her because of what he shared.

Many days passed by then. One night he became very ill. He thought he would die. That very night they had to give him a blood transfusion. He asked me to be with him. I asked the nurse if I could be with him during the transfusion so he wouldn't be alone as he asked. I was vigil over him for several hours until he regained consciousness and he looked at me in the face. He said *"Thanks be to God that you are here. To be by your side is like to be in Heaven."* He asked me to pray for him and then the miracle came – he accepted Jesus Christ as his Lord and Savior.

Personally, that was the happiest night of his life. He made peace with God and was at peace. He no longer feared dying. He found the peace that he was searching for such a long time. In the end, he asked God to forgive him for all the wrong he has done in the world.

Then I asked, *"Do you know what I will do?"*

He replied, *"No, what will you do?"*

I said, *"It has been a long time I have wanted to write a book about the people I met with AIDS."*

He replied, *"I want you to write about me, but I don't want me family to know."* I told him he did not have to worry, his family will never know. Days passed by and he grew worse. Transfusion after transfusion, yet he still grew worse. His fever reached 106 and 107. Others would have died by then but I was always by his side to help him since he did not have any energy for anything. He was very good with me and I was only annoyed three times with him as he had a tremendous temper. He explained to me the reasons why he was incarcerated, always because of his temper. That was the reason he went to jail.

I had already started to write the book and he asked me to write his story. Perhaps tomorrow would serve to help another person so they would not walk the same path as he and end up as he did.

Everything began for Edgar when he was introduced to the famous drug. When he was under the influence of the drug everything appeared more beautiful and rosy colored but the truth was he had no idea where he had been. He was so mixed up with the drugs the drugs were thinking for him. He had no idea what he was doing; he couldn't remember anything.

He told me *"I had no idea I would end up this way – so brutally. But what would we do? I sought it. I went out with women who were addicts. One day, I went out with a friend to buy a pack of cigarettes. My friend entered the store and I waited for him outside. Truly, I do not known what occurred inside that store I only know my friend exited the store with his hands on his head. His head bled. I asked him what happened and he told me the store manager hit him with a club on the head. I never discovered the truth about what really happened since I was outside the store. But I went directly into the store and confronted the man who attacked my friend and asked him why he did that and he replied nastily, "Do you also want me to break your head in?" I exited the store and went directly to my car and pulled out my gun that I always took with me in my car for protection. I returned to the store and grabbed the man who hit my friend and began to hit him until the police came. They handcuffed me and when I turned I noticed my friend had abandoned me. That's what happens when you are mixed up with drugs. You don't have friends. If I did not allow my temper to get the best of me, this would never have happened. Now I am paying the price for both of us; my friend on the outside and me in prison. I am twenty-four years old and dying of AIDS."*

He continues, *"My friend and I were talking when suddenly a corrections officer entered and told us to take our clothes off. We were made to go outside on the patio completely naked by the officer. We were outside for several hours in the severe cold. There was a lot of snow. Two or three days later, I caught pneumonia. It was terrible at night. I had horrible fevers. What made the fevers worse was the yelling and screaming by the other inmates – like they were crazy. Some were raped. For me, it was worse than hell between the fevers and the screaming. I wanted to die. One of the nights when I lay awake unable to sleep but all the others were sound asleep something caught my attention. This wasn't the first time that I heard this noise. Some nights while the rest of the world was sleeping, after mid-night, in one of the cells there were several hooded men in long white tunics. On their chests you could see a big red cross. They would enter one of the cells, grab the prisoner and kick him all over his body. Others would be beaten with sticks. Others with fists until they were almost dead."*

"This seemed like something out of a movie – but it was real. After they killed the prisoner they would say he fell down a stairway. We couldn't say anything for if we did, we never knew when our turn would be next. But the most curious thing was, everyone who died were people of color – blacks or Hispanics. Those they did not kill they left in bad shape. Sometimes, the guards would say they got their injuries fighting other prisoners. Lies upon lies!"

"One night, I became very ill and they had to take me to the hospital due to the pneumonia I contracted. I could not tell the doctors how I contracted the pneumonia for I knew once I returned to the prison they would cut me like a filthy pig. I wanted to avoid any problems. Back to what I was saying, the doctors asked me many questions and conducted several tests. It was then that they told me I contracted AIDS. I thought I would have a heart attack. I told them this cannot be true but unfortunately it was true. How could something like that happen to me? I took a sip of water and regained my composure. Then I told myself it happened to me because I was no one special."

"The doctors entered my quarters and told me they needed to speak with me. They explained everything about AIDS and that they would give me treatment to help me. Sincerely, I had a lot of time to think about it and wondered how I contracted the disease. Everything I have ever done came to my mind – I have played with drugs and with many women who were also drug users. My only desire was to start my life over again."

"It is too late for me, however if someday Josefina publishes her book – this is my one and only wish I ask of God – that others read my story so they do not walk down the path I have taken. I thought life was rosy-colored but how wrong I was! Now that I am here on my deathbed I ask how many others have AIDS. I ask please do not walk down my path – it is not worth the trouble."

"It is now time to go to sleep a bit. Good night Josefina. Tomorrow we will continue the rest; for now, I am too tired. Tomorrow I will continue telling you the rest, right now I feel too weak."

I told him not to worry, sleep peacefully, once and a while I'll check up on him to see how he is doing. The next day I went to see him. I entered his quarters and called out *"Hi Edgar, how do you feel today?"* He replied he felt a little better but only God knows.

He said we would continue where we left off yesterday.

Edgar continued, *"If I had known all of this would happen to me I would have never done all those things – I would have never smoked a pipe or injected drugs or ever been with all those women for none of that was worth the trouble but I have done it and I cannot go back and undo it. Josefina today I feel a little different; I feel stupefied and extreme stomach pain – like a volcano erupting. I don't know what it is but it's like fire that consumes me from the inside."*

He appeared to have a swollen belly and told him so. He replied, *"Yes, the doctors told me they will conduct another test tomorrow to see why but I am already tired of taking so many tests. I am dying and I want them to leave me alone. I don't want them to run anymore tests. I want them to let me die in peace and with dignity."*

I told him not to be nervous, that I would tell the doctors he wished to be left alone that night, not to be bothered. I then went to the doctors and told them.

When I returned to Edgar's quarters to tell him what the doctors said, that since he has been in this condition for several days with several pains, the next day they would take x-rays and other types of tests to see what is causing the terrible stomach pain. The next day, when I returned to work as usual, I felt some intense chills when I moved towards his cell. When I opened the door, I saw him lying on the bed while one of the doctors performed a blood transfusion. He was very pale. I asked the nurse what happened to him. She replied this was the fourth transfusion they gave him today. I could not believe it. In my innermost thoughts I would not have suspected this occurring during the night.

He began to speak to me and asked me to teach him how to pray for he did not know how. After we prayed he looked into my eyes and said *"I cannot go on anymore, I am dying. This stomach pain is the death of me. Help me please."* I told him I could not do anything. He said if he were going to die at least give him something to eat. I replied he knew I could not for the doctors were scheduled to operate on him the following morning. He said, *"I don't want them to operate on me and I will not sign any papers so what are they going to do?"* I asked him why not. He replied, *"Because I'm very afraid, I'm afraid I won't survive the operation."* In the end, I convinced him and he remained asleep, but not for long. In a short while, I heard him scream like a crazy man. I ran to help him. I found him rolling in bed like a serpent. He was crying and screaming. I said," *What is the matter, why are you yelling like that?"* When he turned around, I saw how is abdomen was growing with each passing second. I understood why he screamed so terribly.

He looked at me and asked, *"Why is my stomach so swollen? Please call the doctor or anyone to help me!"* I ran to find the doctor and told him what was happening with Edgar. After the doctor checked him, he told the nurse they must watch over him during the night for he didn't think Edgar would last until morning – his condition was critical but nonetheless they must operate on him in the morning.

Edgar was in bad shape during the night. He wanted to drink water but I would not let him for it could be dangerous. We argued and screamed creating a scandal based from fear all because we would not allow him water. He yelled, *"I am going to die at least let me die happy!"* He said to me, *"Tell everyone to leave here because I want to speak to you alone."* I granted his wish. When everyone left the room he told me *"Help me make a decision; I am very confused."*

I told him he needed to sleep as he had an operation in the morning so he should try to sleep a bit. He replied, *"Ok, you win Josefina."* *"Goodnight Edgar,"* I said.

The next day, they took him to the operation room, but the operation was not a success. There were many complications. They had to leave him in the ICU. Three days passed and he remained in critical condition. When I left work, I would go to visit him, entered the dormitory and saw three people there but not him. Then a Hispanic woman asked me who I was looking for. I told her I was looking for Edgar and she replied Edgar was her son.

She asked me how I know her son and I said that I am Josefina. She said Edgar had told her much about me but also that she believed Edgar would die and I should join her. When I finally saw him, I thought I would have a heart attack. He was so swollen that I could not recognize him. He was in a coma and could not hear me. I took him by the hand and said to him, *"Edgar, I know you can hear me, squeeze my hand."* Immediately, I could feel him squeeze my hand! A tear rolled down his cheek and I knew he could hear me.

He could not answer me, so I kissed him on the cheek and said to him, *"I'll see you tomorrow Edgar."* I felt as if I did not have the energy to even leave his room. Then his mother called me over and said, *"Thank you for taking care of my son. You were his mother when he needed one most."*

She continued, *"You were there, thank you for taking my place. Please forgive all the suffering you had to endure, I should have been there."* I replied *"It was a pleasure to serve for I see Edgar as a brother."* As I left Edgar's room I felt as if the roof of the hospital would collapse upon me.

The next day, Edgar died.

But inside of me I felt a tremendous peace. I knew he was in God's hands. He was in heaven now and did not have to suffer anymore.

Edgar – in your memory I dedicate this part of the book. May God bless your family? You are always in our hearts.

I want my book to be very special because the people written about within are very special to me. I hope they become special to you, the readers, too. You also have a special need for your hearts. I ask when you read the book you become a part of it and I become a part of you. I do not want you to think even for a moment that you are reading science fiction. This my dear friends is not fiction. It is the truth of life and everything I have written within are absolute – as absolute as there is a God in heaven.

Sometimes I ask myself how empty they must feel without having a shoulder to cry on. Without having someone to console them. Perhaps I am the sentimental type but my conscience would eat away at me if I did nothing for them. At the very least to console them and tell them they are not alone. To encourage them as much as possible, giving them the opportunity to feel human, not like lepers. Life is like an hourglass filled with sand – your time is numbered. Perhaps someday my family will be proud of me – well the only things I have are plenty of compassion, comprehension, love and respect. Everyone is loved yet so human they have no hope – also needing spiritual help. We all have the obligation to let everyone know there is a God who loves them no matter what color or nationality they are for God loves everyone equally.

If you recall in the Bible when Mary Magdalene was to be stoned to death, what Jesus said to the multitude, *"He who hath not sinned cast the first stone."* Also, when Moses was in the desert and the people rebelled against Moses and against God – what had happened? God created serpents of fire to kill all the sinners but Jesus said to Moses stand up Moses and lift up your staff. The sky opened and in the sky there was a serpent made of bronze. He said to them, *"Those of us who have been bitten, look! If you have faith and if you repent you will be cured."* Some did not believe and they died. Those who believed were saved. There is a saying that says "with good intentions few words suffice."

Even if you have AIDS look up and see Jesus – your souls will be saved and have eternal life. Jesus is eternal. Sometimes we forget the Ten Commandments. To touch the heart of God we need to be more humble and more responsible. This world is not a festival. We are here to glorify God and to give thanks. He is our Creator. God loves us so much he sent his only son to the world to be crucified, that by this act we would all have eternal life.

All of us, I include myself, have a tendency to do whatever we want not want God wants. That is why we end up thrown to the ground without hope. Today is a great day to start over. Look up to the heavens, the stars, the bright stars, the ocean, the ground. Look all around you and tell me if God is worthy of to be praised. I believe that he is!

Sometimes when we find ourselves in somewhat embarrassing situations who do we call upon? That pride we carry within us does not allow us to give thanks. My God, I believe that one day we will find ourselves and understand. There are many things today we do not understand. We are not paying attention to all the illnesses and many other things.

6. Angel's story

"My name is Angel, I am HIV positive and I am in the Albany Medical Center. They are trying to retain the virus. I never thought I would contract this disease. I acquired it because I was a drug addict and I shared the needles with my friends. That is how I contracted the virus. I hope and pray to God that they find the cure soon. I do not want to die. When the doctors told me I could not believe it. Throughout my life I had gone through many things but I never thought I would end up this way. I was at the verge of death five times but I survived. Now I am blessed for I have lost the battle before and nothing was important to me. I lived in hell; I only thought about the next hit and how I was going to get the money to buy it. I schemed and devised tricks did whatever was necessary in order to get the drugs that I needed. I watched many of my friends die. I hope they are all in heaven. I have gotten to know many good people here in the hospital and I only hope that God and my family forgives me for all the wrong and suffering I have caused them."

"Dearest friend Josefina when you finish this book, I will most likely no longer be in this world but I want you to know where ever I go you will always be in my heart. I say goodbye as a good friend of yours and hopefully, my story will serve to help someone. With respect, I say goodbye to you. Angel."

Tonight was a long night in the hospital like many others, except that all was calm. We had a new patient. I went to take his temperature and he said to me, *"I feel really bad."* I asked him if he wanted me to call the priest and he replied *"I am Catholic."* I replied *"Being Catholic is not enough to go to Heaven when one dies. One must feel very alone to have such an answer."* He then replied *"Yes, I want to go to Heaven."* So I began to tell him about Jesus.

I ask him *"Do you accept Jesus as your personal Savior?"* He replied to me very happily, *"Yes, I do."*

A short while later, one of the nurses told me I had to tend to another patient who tried to commit suicide for the rest of the night. While the patient slept, I took advantage of the time to write. I do this whenever I have the time and also take advantage of moments I am inspired by God. I don't like to be watched over throughout the night by others with crossed arms.

Another night, I have to watch over an elderly man who wanted to get out of bed. The dormitories are kept very cold so I had to find a blanket and remain as guardian the entire night without being able to go to service or even have a cup of coffee lest something happen to the elderly man.

I hoped I would be forgiven for when one has an obligation one has to complete it. At times, I feel very alone when I have to stay the whole night watching over someone. The evening feels so long to me, it feels like it would never end. But, at the end of the night I feel happy because I helped someone. To me, that is the most important thing.

I give thanks to God because he helps me to keep moving forward for there are times that I do not what I would do if he were not a part of me. To me, he helps someone who needs it. It is a major satisfaction for someone who is compassionate. I think we should all treat others as we would like to be treated ourselves. God helps me always to do the right thing. It is 4 a.m. and the old man continues sleeping.

7. John's story

The names of those in this book are the people's actual names. They have given me permission to use their complete names, but I do not dare to for I do not want to upset their families and have them denounce me.

"Hello, my name is John. I am someone who is HIV positive. Everything began when I was eight years old. I lived with my mother, stepfather, my two sisters and a brother. My stepfather and I hated each other to death. One day I became very sick and told my mother that if he did not leave, I would. My mother gave me a suitcase and said to me 'Well leave then, there's the door"

"I left and wandered the streets of New York. Since I was only eight years old, I did whatever I could to survive. I needed to eat and a roof over my head so I began to rob people in order to eat. Later, to get many other things. I moved in with a friend and his family, but they all used drugs so I started using drugs. I smoked marijuana, cocaine, and heroin. I drank beer but was never a drunk. I was so mixed up with drugs I began to shoot up cocaine and heroin at the same time. I destroyed my life. I began to do very bad things – and took the bad road until I ended up in jail."

"I have been locked up for three and a half years in jail but I still have many more to go. I hate everyone around me because they won't get me any drugs. I began to shoot up drugs at twelve years old until I was fifteen"

"When I was fifteen years old, they sent me to prison. I served three and a half years in prison. When I was released, I did not want to live with my

family so I found an apartment somewhere else just for myself. I was in and out of jail constantly. My second home was prison. I knew what I was doing was not good but I did not care about anything at that time"

"I went from one city to the next without staying long in any. Now I am in jail serving seven and a half years to fourteen for a drug problem. I went to court and they denied me [parole]. Now I am aware of all the stupid things I have done – and I detest everything I have done. I have been in jail for three years and I behave the best I can. I am motivated by my conversion to Christianity and I have Jesus Christ in my heart. Now, I no longer have any desire for drugs or to do anything bad. I believe God is with me and he will keep me moving forward. Amen!"

"Now I am in the hospital – Albany Medical Center – because I have the virus. I am HIV positive and I believe with God's help I will get a little better and grow a little stronger at the same time. I never felt free in prison but now that I am a Christian, I feel free because God has given me a new life and I would always honor his name, Amen. I still have four years before I am eligible for parole but I leave it all in God's hands. Well I hope this testimonial helped you Josefina with your book and it would help the youth of today – that life is not a rose garden; life is hard. Farewell, from John – another number in the AIDS casualty count."

8. Gary's story

This part of my book is very special because my family and I took care of Gary all throughout his illness. For us, he was like a brother. We loved him and we suffered greatly until AIDS took him. In his memory, I write this book so that we never forget that Gary was another victim of the monstrosity known as AIDS.

"My name is Gary and I would like to tell you a little bit of my life and how I contracted AIDS. I lived a very disorderly life. My parents were divorced before my first birthday. The court decided I should live with my father. Shortly after he was awarded custody of me, my father could not maintain me let alone take care of me; so my grandmother moved in with us to raise me while my father worked. I remember my father was always working and did everything he could for me, but he was always very busy and did not have time for me. Time went by and my grandmother grew very old. She could no longer raise me so my aunt took me in and raised me in her home."

"I rebelled against her. I felt she was too strict with me. Since my father worked all the time, he was not around to give me discipline. One day I grabbed my things and marched out of the house. I began to do whatever I wanted. As time went on, I got into lots of trouble. The police were looking for me and they finally caught up with me. I was camping in the forest. They confiscated my guns and all of my camping equipment that I had in order to live in. I was a minor, so the court decided not to prosecute. My dad however

was furious with me and decided to teach me a lesson. Through the court, they decided to send me to a reformatory until I reached the appropriate age to know what I wanted to do with my life. They thought that would cause me to change my ways but when everything started to look the darkest; my grandfather came along and took me under his custody. The courts allowed me to be under my grandfather's custody. From that moment on I was under his protection."

"Since I have always been a bit of a wild child, it wasn't difficult for me to find trouble. My drinking problem lead me to even more trouble – and well as many others things. I became a juvenile delinquent. At 16 years old I was a lost cause. But my grandfather loved me and always remained positive. He always believed that someday I would change my ways. He loved me with all his heart and continued helping me. Taking care of me no matter what anyone said about me. He was always there. It didn't matter what time of day or day of the week. After 14 years of crime and problems, my grandfather began to grow weak. His heart could no longer take the strain my trouble brought and he died."

"My life changed overnight. I found myself alone and find a way to support myself. To find a place to live without having anyone to turn to. I always depended on him. Now I was alone and no idea what to do. In the darkness of my room I thought my life was over. I was wrong."

"This of course, was the start of all my troubles. I was so disoriented I returned to drugs and became addicted to cocaine, heroin and alcohol. I was hooked to the injections and had a habit of more than $300 a day. After a while I lost my job. Doing such bad things I couldn't concentrate on it. Instead, without my realizing it, I began committing armed robbery and other criminal activity. In the end, I was arrested and sentenced to jail."

"When I entered the correctional system, they took me to the hospital. That's when I realized I was infected with the HIV virus. Things were not looking the way I imagined, but I had to live with it for the rest of my life. Then one day, someone spoke to me about someone who loved me. I replied I had no one. That's when I was introduced to Jesus Christ and I asked him to be my Lord and Savior. Now I no longer fear anyone or anything since I have dedicated my life to God. Things appeared different and better."

"I spent the majority of my time studying the Bible – studying the word of the Lord. I learned and grew in the grace of our Lord, Jesus Christ. My life was renewed thanks to God. I had three people who loved me above all others – I had the Father, the Son and the Holy Spirit. I began to talk to other prisoners about Christ and how he changed my life. Because the fruit of the spirit is love, peace, happiness and longer suffering gentleness, better conditions, faith, humility. Because the fruit of the spirit is good."

"Never go back because the price of sin is death. The death that separates us from God. Since the day I gave myself to Jesus Christ my life has become better. I study the Bible and that helps me understand the word of God. He is the one who helps me to continue forward during the hard times of my life. Sometimes I have difficult moments; I don't want to accept I have AIDS, but Jesus gives me strength to continue onward. He comforts me when I am alone and depressed. I give him thanks because he never turned his back on me. When I needed him most, he was there. For the grace of God I live day to day and he gives me strength to keep going. I live with the promises that he has given me. May god use this testimonial for his glory, Amen."

"This is a poem I wrote for people with HIV:

1. *Your bodies are like rigid trees*
2. *Your lips are like two discolored petals*
3. *Your arms are like branches from an arid tree*
4. *Your veins like dried roots*
5. *Your eyes like two holes without end*
6. *Your legs seem are like dried splinters*
7. *Your cheeks seem like two unripe apples*
8. *Your ears look like used glue*
9. *Your hair like a tree when the leaves have fallen*
10. *Your nails look like a bowl of dried fruit*
11. *Your color like olives*
12. *Your scent like a turbulent ocean*
13. *Your muscles look like steel bars*
14. *Your stomach is like an active volcano*
15. *Your illness like the gateway to the hells of poison*

"With all my love and all of my affection I dedicate this poem to all the people that I love so much. I love all of those people who suffer this terrible illness because they are very special to me – because they have courage to fight a battle that is already lost. I am with you and Jesus is with you to the end, Amen."

Today was a particularly appreciated day for me for we had two days off from work and I had time to think. I never stop thinking mind you, even when I am sleeping. My brain seems to be restless for I have so much on my mind – my family, my patients.

Sometimes I think if there is something that we want to do and it is within our hearts I think we should do them. And we should deprive ourselves for it is never easy to reach our goals. We should have confidence in ourselves. Often I think of all these people who never had the opportunity to be someone in their lives. I feel I am very fortunate for God is always nearby me and helps me get out many situations I do not understand. I give thanks to God for he is always near me and protects me.

He gave me an opportunity and I want to help those who need me. I only ask him to give me strength to keep going and help all those that I can. Time, for me, is like gold and diamonds. Many people write about AIDS – how to avoid it; how to detect it; and so much more. Doctors talk among themselves, we should be doing this and that and the other. But nobody takes heed. They know. So many of them believe they do. In reality, or how they think, the doctors do not have time for their patients.

The patients are human beings and have feelings; they are not machines. They think about how many more experiments will be performed on them. When someone gets close to them you begin to understand them and care about them. They appreciate you with all their hearts.

Today, the jails are full of prisoners that have AIDS. But of course, that is a fact of very little importance to anyone. The majority of them are homosexuals, the rest are drug addicts. In the jail, many things occur that no one knows about. Only those who are there know. The prisoners told me everything that occurs in jail. It seems incredible but what they tell me is true. The people who are in jail and have AIDS suffer greatly but they receive no treatment. Apparently, that costs the state too much money and to the state, having AIDS is the prisoners' problem. I have watched them die for lack of medical attention. The infirmary at the jail might as well be a slaughterhouse. The people who work within them are butchers.

They mistreat them, and some are spat on and insulted like dogs. In truth, for someone to have AIDS is like those in ancient times to have leprosy. This is a problem we must all deal with and we should help them. Even they themselves cannot comprehend what is happening to them. I think that in some way we should help them resolve this tremendous problem.

We do not have much time. If those who are in jail are released into the street, there would be many more people with AIDS. Many of the prisoners go by a long time without the company of women. Others want revenge and spread AIDS into the street like candy. Innocent people will pay for what the prisoners have done. It is a terrible tragedy and I cannot see the solution to this monster that is terminating many of our loved ones.

I wish to help them but I cannot do it alone. We need many volunteers for the battle will be long and laborious. I have hoped that someday with God's help we could do something for them.

God has given me the gift of love for those who others despise. They are human beings and have feelings like all of us. Sometimes I wonder who we would react if we were in their place? Perhaps we would understand them better however since we are not in their place we could never understand.

Sometimes I think we are too egotistical. Instead of criticizing them we should learn more about AIDS. That way we could help them rather than judge them.

During the time I worked with them I have seen families abandoned the patients like dogs in the hospital and that broke my heart. So I think if they knew more about AIDS they would not abandon them. The majority of us guide ourselves by what appears beautiful; and some of us pay for that with our lives.

Some lose their lives so they do not want to go through all the suffering. Those that survive, the only thing they have left is to wait for death to come to them as soon as possible. They need a great deal of moral support as well as love and compassion. Knowledge that they are not alone would brighten their lives. They feel like they are useless and a burden. But that is not true! I think they are people who need a great deal of love. At times, I wish I could express everything I feel about them.

9. Emilio's story

Emilio was a very good patient, but like everyone else was HIV positive and was becoming blind; a consequence of the same illness. Emilio and I spoke frequently but he was Hispanic and spoke Spanish so we practiced the language. Every day I helped him eat or go to the bathroom as he could not see anything due to his HIV. I asked him if he didn't mind being included in my book. He replied he didn't mind at all – what would I like to know?

"The truth," I said, *"about how you came to contract AIDS … how you ended up in such a big mess?"* He responded, *"I do not even know how I got here but I got started as many other young people my age have – I got involved in extremes I do not even know how I did. I asked God to forgive me of all wrong-doing I have done. Now I am paying the consequences for all I have done. But let's continue with the story as I begun to tell you. I started by fooling around with friends. They would say 'come over here man, don't be scared; try it – no one has died from just trying it.' They insisted so much that I agreed and before I knew it I was in an alley with no way out."*

"I asked God to help me. I don't know how I am going to change my life but as I was telling you I found myself robbing in order to pay for my vices. Believe me, my vices were not cheap! Drugs, women, I've done it all. Things even I cannot believe. Had I been normal, I would never have done. When they arrested me and placed me in jail I had a lot of time to think

about everything I had done and repented what I had become but it was too late to go back."

"I had to take the first step and that was jail. In jail I had a lot of time to think and I decided to get away from drugs and clean up my internal system. But the temptation was too great – alas the prisoners sold drugs in jail."

"I hope you are not getting bored with everything I am telling you?"

I replied, *"Do not worry and please continue; I am not bored. Honestly, when the public reads my book, I want them to know it is really you and not me who is recanting your tale. It is part of your life."*

"I ask God to give me strength to keep moving forward," continued Emilio, *"and able to die with dignity."*

Emilio asked me to pray with him. I replied, *"As you wish Emilio."* After we prayed he felt much better. He asked Christ to enter his heart and give him eternal life. He gave his heart and his soul to our Lord and Savior Jesus Christ. Today Emilio became a Christian and while he has HIV he also has Jesus. He will be the one who will help in during his final days so his life will be much more pleasant.

He told me, *"If I told you something would you write it in your book?"* I replied, *"Of course."*

Emilio said, *"I implore you, please do not commit the same mistakes I have committed. Sometimes we want to be manly and do not want to say to our friends that you no longer see where this road takes you. I had wished I could go back but alas it is already too late. I can no longer go back but I can warn others they still have time and implore them to please do not follow my example. I know what I am talking about for now I am paying the price and it was not worthwhile."*

"I am not the only one paying for it – my family is as well. They know that I am dying and that consumes them. My wife will be a widow and my daughter fatherless. To tell me this does not hurt rips my heart apart just to think about it. I wish to live the remainder of my life making my family happy and asking God to illuminate my path every day. The path ahead of me is horrible. After I am released from the hospital they will send me directly to jail. As just desserts, I will die in jail like a dog. If this is not

suffering, then I do not know what is. I would like to give you more over my testimony but I have nothing left. Only to say whoever plays with fire will get burned. And you must pay for your consequences."

"I have nothing left to say and I give thanks to God for sending me Josefina for she has helped me greatly. May the Lord bless her for all she has done for me? I will return to jail and let that be the will of God. In jail, we are like lepers the other prisoners do not even wish to look at us. I think I need to resign for now and keep moving forward for lives moves on. I hope that one day you and I will see each other again, God only knows."

Today is like any other day at my job with much work to do and little time to think about other more important things, like, for instance, in the people who have so much fear contracting AIDS, but if it is easier to contract tuberculosis or hepatitis rather than HIV and AIDS without understanding why people do not fear of other diseases that are more contagious than AIDS?

My head spins and I cannot achieve understanding of anything. People have more fear of what they see than what they don't see. It should be the opposite. I believe this is something psychological for this has no explanation. None for the least or at least none I can find. I would like to be able to tell these people that HIV is not leprosy. It seems like the whole world is in a panic and they cannot think for themselves. It is a real shame that instead of thinking with their hearts they think with their feet.

If we use our brains we could comprehend that these people who have HIV need us and many have no one that loves them and that is not right! Who are we to judge anyone? I give thanks to God for he has a great deal of patience with us. He gave us the commandment to love one another for the fellowship of mankind is most important even though it doesn't appear that way to us.

If we do not have love for ourselves how can we have love for other people? The love of others that we truly need? Sometimes it is difficult to relate to someone who is dying because we are not in their place but I would like to know how we would react if it were us in their place. I cannot make my point any clearer.

I ask God to help me and keep giving me health for as long as I have health I will continue helping these kinds of people. Now is when they need us the most for they cannot fight for themselves. Sometimes we are too egotistical for we only think of ourselves. That is a shame for within us all we carry someone who if we wanted could be amazing but our pride and our dignity and many other things are in the way. I know for sure that if my friends knew that I work with people that have AIDS they would probably never speak to me again. But for me, the most important is to make people who need happiness happy – the rest does not matter.

We will never get anywhere once we are sick and broke unless we have friends. It may sound silly but it is true. I know from experience. Every day I go to work my heart breaks as I see more and more people in need of love and compassion. They feel; so alone, some of them tell me their story and it brings me such sadness for after so much suffering they end up here to die like dogs and without anyone to love them.

But there is a God, so big and each one of us can pick up what is planted. That is why I do everything I can for them and even more but alas one person alone cannot do it all. She needs more people to help her. The only thing I earn is the feeling of happiness that they know I have given them the best I can and I appreciate it with all my heart.

Sometimes I ask God to perform miracles and that they convert. In truth, God is all powerful and can create and destroy. I give him thanks for all the miracles he performed in my life. But for the grace of God I could have ended up like anyone of them. Who knows? Only God knows. I always ask him on behalf of these needy people and if I do something incorrect I ask for his forgiveness for I have done it without bad intentions and made errors, we all are humans. Even though some of the mistakes we make are more painful and sad than others, but there is something called repent.

10. Victor's story

H i, what is your name? – *"My name is Victor"* - Victor is Hispanic, like the majority of the patients we have here at this hospital. He just got admitted to the hospital like an hour ago. He is HIV positive and has an infection on his brain. His head hurts a lot; he is a little confused and speaks very little English.

"Hi Victor, I'm the nurse assistant and I'll be the one taking care of you at night if you ever need anything. My name is Josefina. Victor, I'm going to ask you a couple of questions that are very personal and particular. I'm writing a book about people that has AIDS, and I would like you to help me – that is, if you don't mind. I would like you to tell me how did you became HIV positive." He said, *"I don't know where to start."*

"Start from the beginning and don't get nervous, that is the most important thing."

"I was born at the Bronx; I don't know if you know about that community, it's where I spent all my life and where the majority of the Hispanics live in. Everybody is very poor and you know when you are poor and there is no money you start having problems at home. I always saw people fight because they didn't had money to feed their children, or the owners of the house would come in and kick a family out of their house leaving them with no place to live, no food. Well, what can I say? It truly is very hard. When I saw and heard those things it really horrified me the idea of that happening to me one day. So everyday when I got up I told to

myself. "Where would I start today?" But one day, we started lacking things at home and we needed to find money one way or the other. My friends and I started stealing. Trying to figure out what we could take and sell in order to be able to eat. If you haven't experience that, you don't know how hard it is. It's hard to do things you don't want to do but there is not other alternative."

"I tried to find a job but I don't know how to write or read, I'm illiterate and no one wants to hire somebody like that, nobody wanted to give me an opportunity. By that time I was going through a lot of misery and you become very rough. Many times they offered me marijuana and I said no. Then they called me a coward, a faggot, etc. One time I said "yes, but only a little bit" and that's how I started, first time a little bit then more and more. I got hooked. I was now stealing to support my addiction not because I needed things. I had to get out and do things I didn't wanted to do. It was all a catastrophe and it was getting worse and worse. My family didn't know what was going on with me, they were all worried about me, and they saw I was getting worse. I didn't want them to suffer so I kept it all from them. Many times I wished I died, I disgusted myself. There was always the next day and I thought everything was going to end. How wrong was I, it all looked like it had no ending. One day I got really sick. My family was very scared, they thought I was going to die and when everything was over I had no idea what had happened to me."

"After I got better, I told my friends I wanted to get out of it, I couldn't continue doing those things because they were wrong and I couldn't continue that way. My friends put a lot of peer pressure on me. They told me to smoke pot again, to not leave everything for a silly thing and that I would feel better. They told me I didn't need any money, they were going to give me the pot for free. I went back to stealing again and many other things, anything I needed to do to get drugs. Time kept passing by and every day I did worst things, everyday I needed more things to buy more and more drugs. Drugs were more expensive also. My life was a tragedy, every time I look back I wish somebody would have told me what was going to happen to me and that what I was doing was wrong. I never wanted to listen to *anybody, I wanted to keep doing thins my way and because of that, I am what I have become today."*

"One day I did something extremely bad and I'm still paying for it today. The police got me and now I'm in jail paying for it. It is not worth it; because of drugs and women I am now HIV positive. I don't know what else can happen to me. I can't blame anybody but me; I am harvesting what I've planted. It is normal; a person who plants good seeds at the end gets what he planted. From Jail to the hospital, that's my life. I would like to tell you more things but some stuff I would like to keep for myself, some things are very private."

"It's fine Victor, I don't want you to feel pressure."

"I feel much better now; I have taken a big pressure out of my life and that knot I had on my chest for a long time. I give God thanks because I know He is the one who sent you. Now that I'm here I hope I can have some peace and calm. All through these years I haven't found a person so kind and good with me. Are you sure you are not an angel that came from heaven?"

-   "No Victor, I'm not an angel. But perhaps you would like to know why I am different; if you want I can share it with you."

"Yes, I would like to know. Must be something good, I can see it in your eyes. Why are you crying Josefina? I didn't want to offend you."

-   "No, its nothing. I just want to thank God. He put me in your path."

-   "I'm thankful too. Josefina, would you care if I call you Fina?"

-   "No Victor, I don't mind at all, that's how my family calls me."

-   "I would like you to tell me what is it that you have that makes you different."

-   "Let me tell you, I am a Christian, that means I am under Jesus Christ's protection. Want I want to tell you is that four years ago I accepted Jesus Christ in my heart and I asked him to forgive all the sins I had committed and to give me eternal life."

"And what happened? Did He listen?"

"Yes Victor, Jesus entered my life and gave me eternal life. When I die, I will go to heaven with him. Since then I have dedicated my life to let people know there is a remedy and his name is Jesus Christ. He is the only one that can change our lives."

"Fina, I want you to share that Jesus you have."

"-Of course I can Victor; we can be brothers in faith. Well Victor, now that you have Jesus in your heart you need to try to sleep. We'll continue talking some other time, now its time for you to go rest or the medicine they gave you is not going to have any effect on you."

"Ok sister, as you wish."

"-Ok Victor, see you later."

This is a new day for Victor; I'm going to go check how he feels.

"Hi Victor, how are you feeling today?"

"Not so good, they have done so many tests on me, my whole body hurts."

"What do you have other than HIV?"

"I don't know, they took some liquid from my spine and I can hardly move."

"It is normal that your back hurts Victor, and you will be in pain for a couple more days."

"I need a cigarette Fina."

"I don't smoke but I will try to find you one."

Half hour after I came back with the cigarettes.

"What do you think Victor, I find you the cigarettes!"

"I'm so happy Fina, What a joy to be able to smoke a cigarette, thank you Fina for being so good with me. May God always bless you and protect you."

"Do you have anything else you want to share with me for my book?"

"Yes, there's something else."

"Ok Victor, I'm listening."

"I wish I could go back and start all over again. I know is impossible, please forgive me Fina, but today I'm very depressed and I don't know why. I'm so afraid; the doctors have been doing too many medical experiments on me. They pinch me everywhere and can't find my veins. I don't know what to do, I'm getting desperate."

"Now that I'm here you can talk to me Victor."

"Today a Social Worker came and told me that he wanted to talk to all of us. They had a meeting for everybody who is HIV positive. They wanted us

to tell them how do we feel knowing we are living with AIDS and knowing we are going to die soon. I asked him how he would feel if it was him living with AIDS. He never answered my question. They believe by talking to us we are going to feel better. They are only making us feel worse."

"Victor, if you want we can continue other day."

"No, I want to talk with you and tell you how I feel. I'm comfortable with you. When they ask me all those questions I feel trapped, nowhere to go. But you Fina, you understand us; you live with us every day, cry and suffer with us. You console us, clean us up, and feed us. We trust you, they are so cold and they don't care about us. They don't even care how we feel; they just want to use us as lab rats. I feel like I'm in a cage waiting for the next experiment."

"Don't get nervous Victor; everything is going to be ok. All you need to do is tell them you don't want to talk to them when they come back. They can't make you talk to them. Problem solved, ok?"

"I need something to drink Josefina, I'm really thirsty."

"I'll get you something right away, but promise me you will calm down."

"I need something for the pain Fina."

"Ok Victor, no problem, but after that you will go to sleep, ok?"

"Yes, I promise."

Victor stayed with us at the hospital for at least a month. He got much better, he didn't have so many headaches and he looked like he was feeling better. They told him he was being released from the hospital but he didn't want to go back to prison. Three days after I got back to work and he wasn't there anymore, he was sent back to jail. I missed him for some time. I thought that maybe now he was feeling better and was happy.

Two weeks later, I was with a patient when a nurse called me and told me to get room 422 ready. We had an admission. I told her that I would do it right away; I went and took all the stuff to get the room ready. Half hour later they had a patient there. I went to get my stuff to take his blood pressure, his pulse etc.

What a surprise when I went to the room and it was Victor on the bed. He had tubes in his body and was ready to receive a blood transfusion. I asked him how he was doing and he told me he felt really sick and thought he would die that night. I told him not to say those things, but he told me he didn't feel good and he knew there was nothing he could do. I asked him how were things going for him and he said that things were not that bad but kept saying he wanted to die to finally rest in peace. He asked me if I remember the last time he was there, how can I forget? I said. He told me that when he was here last time, they took liquid from his spine five times and now he can't walk, move the right side of his body or see through his right eye.

"You tell me what this people have done with me. I'm much worst now than when I came the first time. Please pray for me, I don't know what's going to happen with me."

"If I can help you Victor, please let me know. You have to be patient; God didn't create the world in one day. Some day we will find the answer to all of this. Doctors don't do miracles, but God does. He has the remedy to cure all illnesses. What happens is that we never want to pay any attention; we want to do as we feel and that's not right."

A couple of days later they released Victor. All nights are the same here, always talking about suffering. Sometimes I go to the bathroom and start crying until I don't have anymore tears. It is so hard to see them die little by little and I can't do anything. When I'm done crying I just come out of the bathroom like nothing happened. I don't want them to notice I suffer too. Some patients know me very well and they notice, they say to me: *"God bless you for sharing our pain and our loneliness, don't worry, we will see each other at heaven and enjoy all this moments."* That is the only thing that makes me happy, the ability to help them all I can. Sometimes it is terrible; I wish I didn't have to be here.

All I see every day is dead people and more dead people, I wish I could disappear. I can't let myself feel that way; nobody knows what it is to feel this way all the time. We get patients, we take care of them, they leave and then come back. One day they come back and can't leave anymore, they are out of energy. They stay here and I see them die gradually. At the end they all leave. It is terrible to live like this, we get used to them and they start being part of you; when they die is like you are having a bad dream. You see them so skinny, pale and rigid. They remind me of Hitler's prisoners, all skin and bones. You can imagine what is to have that on your mind. In this case, Hitler is not the enemy. This one is worst because it's like it's never going to end. I wish I could describe it better but can't, there is no other way than this. When the moment arrives and they die, I see them dead in their beds and I feel like my heart is going to explode in pain. When one of them dies it's like having a thorn in your heart.

11. Jose's story

It was a night like every other when the phone rang. They called me and told me there was an admission for the N5 room. I let the nurse know, she took the patients details and I got the room ready for the new patient. An hour later they got him in the room, I took his blood pressure and pulse. I asked him what was his name and he said Jose. He told me that he didn't felt good at all. He had headaches and stomach pains. I told him the nurse would give him the medicine to make him feel better. After some time went by, I heard screaming and went back to check who was it. The screaming came from Jose's room; he told me he was still waiting for the nurse to come give him something for the pain. I went to look for the nurse and when I found her she told me she had already gave him a morphine shot.

I went back to Jose's room, who was still screaming, and told him what the nurse had told me. He insisted that she hadn't given him anything, so I called the nurse again and told her. She got really mad and went to call the doctor. The nurse told the doctor about it and he told her to give him another shot. *"But I gave him one shot 15 minutes ago,"* she said. But the doctor told her to give him the shot anyway. The nurse gave him the morphine and 20 minutes later he was already screaming again.

I went to his room to find out what was going on and he told me the same thing, the nurse hasn't given me anything. I told him it's wasn't true, I saw when the nurse gave him the shot. I asked him to just go to sleep and rest a little. He looked at me with so much pain in his eyes.

All of the sudden two big tears came from his yes and he said, *"Ok, I'll do whatever you want me to do."* I told him, *"Good night, sweet dreams,"* and he fell asleep like a baby. I thought to myself, thank God he is asleep already; he is in so much pain. I wish I could express to him all the love and compassion I feel for him but at this moment the pain he feels can't let him realize it. What he can see is the difference between a person that cares and worries about him with love, not with disgust like many people look at them here. It's like they are lepers or a different thing. There is something very special about Jose, I see him as my brother and that makes me suffer a lot because I would like to help him and treat him like he is really my brother. His HIV is attacking his brain; night after night I have cared and prayed with him. I have asked God to liberate him from the horrible pain in his head. I know He heard me, after five minutes of praying he falls asleep like a little boy without knowing that God has answered my prayers. I just gave God thanks for being so good to me.

Jose wasn't able to eat, nothing would hold in his stomach and everything he ate he threw up. Sometimes I gave him juice so he had something in his stomach. When his headache starts I bring him a cold towel to help him feel better and be able to relax. After, I massage his temples and tell him everything is going to be alright. He would tell me he knew everything was going to be alright but he needed to be more patient. I told him that faith would move mountains. It's very complicated to have to talk with somebody who is dying because you really don't know what to tell them. With love, affection and God's grace, everything is possible.

Jose stayed at the hospital for two more months. I've seen him when he was really sad, when he was better and when he almost died. HIV positive patients have no future, they are living like they are dead, and all they have to look for is the day they get to die. It is not easy, how can we be so cold? I think we should be more humanitarian and have more compassion with each other. In God's eyes, we are all equal, we like it or not we all are brothers and sisters. I don't know what else to do for you to have compassion. I ask God everyday to give me strength to continue helping these people, people like Jose and many others that suffer from this illness.

Jose was feeling really sick; we thought he was going to die. I've never seen him that bad. He was throwing up and in a lot of pain. I went to talk to him, they didn't let the nurses went in and help him. When I went in he was screaming in Spanish and nobody understood him. I asked him to please calm down and he replied, *"I want to die, this pain is like having your brain on fire, it feels like something is cutting my brain in little pieces."* I told him to calm down, the medicine was coming. The nurse gave him a morphine shot but in 15 minutes he was already screaming again. He told me to please give him more morphine. The nurse refused to give him more and told him he needed to wait three hours to get another shot.

Jose turned over his body to the window and told her, *"Look at how I get this resolved right now, I'm sorry but I can take this anymore, I'm going to jump out the window."* I reacted quickly and before he jumped I grabbed his waist and pulled him back. He fell on top of me, causing me damages in my shoulder and leg. I thank God he is alive, he hurt his eye with the corner of the table but other than that he is fine. The nurse ran back when she heard me screaming. There were five police officers at the door and none of them helped me get up. They were all looking, but none of them did anything to help with the situation. I was under Jose and he was unconscious. They just kept looking at us like nothing was happening. The nurses came in and helped me get up from the floor.

When I went out of the room the police officers asked me: *"Why didn't you let him jump out the window?"* I responded: *"You think because he is HIV positive he doesn't have the right to live? Why didn't you help me?"*

They told me they didn't want to get infected with HIV.

I looked at them with disgust and told them: *"You never know if we would see if each other again and you will be the patient."*

When I got into the bathroom I asked God forgiveness because I looked at them with disgust. Then I understood that with just the mention of the word HIV they were terrified to the point they didn't wanted to get inside the room. When people hear this word, they don't know what to do and when someone is terrified, they don't understand what you are telling them, even if it is in their own language. That's one the reasons I'm writing this book, so people understand that you don't get AIDS by touching someone.

Jose stayed at the hospital at least two more months and kept getting better. Today, he is much better, still living with HIV. The time came for him to go back to prison. The day before it, I went and talked to him about dedicating his life to be a Jesus Christ servant. He told me he believes in God so I asked him to pray. I asked him to pray to God to be his savior and to forgive all his sins, to have God get into his heart and give him eternal life so when he dies, he goes to heaven. I told him I would see him in there someday and we would remember this night and he would not suffer more, under God's grace, we are all perfect. Next day when I came back to work he was no longer there. Five months later his family contacted me to let me know he died. More pain for my heart, another thorn in my soul. AIDS had won another battle.

Tonight has been fairly calm, and looks like it's going to go fine. I feel a little depressed. I haven't been able to talk to anybody because the patients we have are all in a bad stage. I prayed today for a new patient I can talk to and tell him how much Jesus loves him. God has listened to me; they just called and told us they are bringing a new patient. I'm going to get the room ready for when he arrives. He only speaks Spanish. I'm the only one who speaks Spanish here; nobody understands what he is saying so I need to serve as interpreter. He is very scared, doctors talk to him and he only moves his head, he is trying to tell them he doesn't understand. He is trying to tell the doctors what he is feeling in Spanish but the doctors don't understand him. I asked him what was wrong and he told me his head hurt and so did his shoulder. I looked at his shoulder and noticed he had a surgery wound and it was still tender. This was causing a lot of pain but nobody understood how or why. Nobody understood him; at least I was there to help.

I served as interpreter at the hospital due to the fact that I speak English, Spanish and Italian. I asked him if he knew who Jesus was and he told me that he thought so. I asked him if he wanted me to show him how to pray, he converted into a Christian and accepted Jesus Christ in his heart. I called him "brother in faith" and he smiled at me. I told him he needed to learn how to pray and ask God to help him with his illness because it is really hard to always be thinking about how much time you have to live. I asked him if he knew how was in heaven and he told me he knew about heaven that he had seen it in his dreams. I asked him to tell me how it was. "It's a beautiful city, very clean. The streets are pure gold and it sparkles like a diamond."

After that he got better and was sent home. That was the last time I saw him. But he is no longer with us; he also lost the battle to AIDS. Now he is another one AIDS has taken, another battle AIDS has won.

12. Jose's story (a different Jose)

This is another night and another patient. His name is Jose, he is also Hispanic. I met him in November; he has two girls and a boy. He looks like he has suffered a lot. He stayed here for a month and was very sick. He had very high fevers and could hardly talk. His fevers cause him to be delirious and we couldn't understand what he was saying. Many nights after I did my rounds I went to see him, he felt really lonely.

Of course, who wouldn't be depressed knowing you are going to die? Nobody feels good knowing they are going to die. Thank God I always have time for him and that helps him a lot and helps his morale.

During the time he was here he behaved very good, didn't cause us any problems. At first he was rough and didn't want to make any friends, but very soon we became friends. I went to see him every day and talked with him; made me feel good, those moments were very important for him, it was good for him to felt he had someone to talk with.

One day he got very sick and I went to see him. I asked him what was wrong and he said, *"I don't know, but I feel really bad"*. He had really high fevers and was delirious again. I told him I was thinking about talking with him about something very important. He asked me what that was. I explained to him I was a Christian and I wanted him to convert to into a Christian. He told me he didn't knew how to and I told him that all he needed was to say a little payer and ask Jesus Christ to forgive all his sins and He would enter in his heart. He told me he wanted to do that so I helped him pray and he accepted Jesus Christ in his heart and he is now a Christian, he has Jesus in his heart. He will never be alone now.

It is hard to know how to behave like a Christian in jail, people will laugh at you. But God is there with us, we need to fear no one. Jose was with us for some time, he felt this time was very short. He felt very happy between us. When it was time for him to leave he didn't wanted to, he had to go back to jail. I can't blame him, who wants to go back to jail? Especially when you have AIDS, the other prisoners treat you really badly. It is really bad knowing you are going to die while at jail. I think it is horrible to just think when is it going to happen? That moment seems it would take forever. I can't even begin to think about it, I feel really bad just to think about it. It is not my fault he is sick, what I have is the responsibility of taking care of him. It wouldn't be very humanitarian of me not to think this way.

Jose and I have talked about many things, especially about his testimony. I need all the information I can get from him for my book. I asked God to help me and give him strength. He wants me to put his name on my book and that makes me happy. At least he is not ashamed about having AIDS. There is nothing to be ashamed of, this is an illness. An illness that consumes your body like fire consumes a building. Jose is willing to give me his testimony. He told me that as soon as they remove all his tubes he would be giving me his testimony.

Thank God for people like him, they made a lot of things possible. When I got to my job today I found my friend extremely worried, he has had really high fevers throughout the day and the night. I thought it was going to be his last night and so did everyone else. Thank God his fevers went down and he looked like he was doing much better. When dawn came, he couldn't remember anything of the night before. He was delirious all night long due to the high fevers. We talked for some time and he looked better. The next couple of days made him worry even more.

Every time he gets into the hospital, he stays for two weeks and then it's back to jail, still sick. I don't know why they do that. One day will have the answer to all these questions, the things I see doctors do to him make no sense at all. Medicine doesn't make miracles happen, but God does. Every day I see God's hand in and for me, that's something very special. I always tell Jose, because he is a Christian like me, that if God wasn't real, I don't know where we would be with all the things we have to deal with everyday.

Having to fight this illness is not a fun thing, it is something very serious; we need to have a lot of understanding, love and patience because it becomes part of you and that is very hard. Only someone with a big heart can understand, you have to give yourself entirely. I'm happy, people like Jose is grateful that I help him every day and it shows. They see what I do is with love, not with disgust or revulsion. I do it with much love and understanding and that is the only thing we can do for them. Jose is one of many patients I take care at the hospital; many of them die in my hands and it's very sad.

It's really hard, you take care of them and you are fond of them and then they die. I have to put their bodies in a plastic bag and say goodbye forever. I will never see them again, is their last day of suffering and their last ride. There's nothing pleasant about going through this different situations. You spent your nights giving them comfort like you are like their mother, and you feel this emptiness inside your heart you can't even begin to imagine. They belong to their mothers, but I'm the one in that place, their mothers are not available at those moments. It is hard not to get fond of them, and when they ask for a hug not to give it to them or just sit and listen to them when they are in pain or depressed. I feel really bad I can't do anything else for them. I am only one person and I can't do anymore. I'm mentally and physically exhausted with all this suffering. God is always with me and he gives me strength to continue, He helps me with my pain.

Jose's presence makes me remember all the patients that are here. They all are different, but at the same time they all have the same thing in common, HIV positive. That keeps them united; believe it or not they all have the same symptoms. Jose makes me aware of how he is feeling and that helps me help the other patients. They all are so scared and desperate they can become violent sometimes.

I need to be very careful with them, but at the same time let them know I care for them. At the end you get close to them, they let you get close to them, and that is an honor for me. They share things with you they won't even share with ministers. You become the confessional. They get used to you and dependant on you, this makes it easier for them, you become part of them and share they good moments as well as the bad ones. But, until you get to that point you really have to work with them. Some of them are very private, which makes it impossible to talk to them. I've never had that problem, but I have seen the problems the other nurses had with patients before. Patients don't really share anything with the other nurses, nurses only see them as sick people and that's it. I see them as sick souls asking for help, and that is the most important thing for me.

I'm not perfect, but I like to help them and offer them my company. The company that they lack so much and I can offer since they trust me. They know I would never betray them. I sometimes feel like them, maybe because we are so close. Before Jose left, he told me he would write to me, he wants to continue being my friend not only my patient. I understand him; he is a very good person. Sometimes I feel like I'm not myself, all this pain, all this suffering, why and for what? It's not easy living with HIV.

When people hear that word they run away scared. If we all pay a little bit more attention we would be able to understand what this illness is about. Maybe that would make us think in a different way. How are we going to change our mind if it's easier to just keep them away? It's not fair, they are human beings too and we never know if we can become one of them. Only God knows what they go through. Their bodies consume itself like a tree you cut and it starts dying little by little until you have nothing left. The only difference is that those are trees and these are human beings. We should treat them like human beings. It is not easy for them or for me to explain to people that in the last 24 hours the only thing they did was think about when they are going to die.

The only thing we can do is give them courage so they can continue and keep thinking positively. The only thing they have left is pray to God to cure them or to help them die sooner before all the suffering. It is very painful to find yourself in this situation. We should always put ourselves in somebody else's situation to find out how they feel. We should try to feel like they do, this way we would be able to understand them. The only thing I can say is that I'm able to understand them very well because I live and spend time with them. I pray to God to give me the strength and the health to continue doing the job that I love. They are part of me and I'm part of them. It's really painful when you have to separate one part from the other; it's not the same anymore.

13. The woman

I met a lady who is not a patient here, and she told me how she got infected with HIV. She told me she had a very good life and had whatever she wanted. She went to the most luxurious places, had a lot of fun all the time and lived life to the fullest everyday. She was free, wasn't attached to anyone, so she did what she wanted. But at the end, all of the things that looked beautiful were over and all she had were shadows and dreams. Everything that used to be happiness was now pain. There is no time to laugh anymore, now everything is very serious.

She always told me, *"I'm paying the price now. It was all vanity, it all looked very beautiful, but it wasn't. How wrong was I? We now need to live realistically; we don't have any other alternative. Now we don't have much were to choose from, hard to believe but true. Everything that we enjoyed thinking it was good it's really not and now we pay the consequences. It's not easy, when we do it we don't stop and think about if it's right or wrong."*

This is the third time she has been here. She looks so nice, I really like her. Every time I go see her she receives me with a smile on her lips. She has accepted very well the fact that she has AIDS. It is not easy to accept the reality she lives in, knowing you are dying sooner or later but don't know really when. I don't think a lot of people would know how to overcome the sadness of being sick with this illness. She is a very strong woman, she herself gives her the courage to continue and that's not an easy thing to do, not everybody can do it. I try to stay in contact with her as much as I can, I love her very much. I have her in my heart like every other person that suffers here. I share that lonely suffering they all have deep inside that has no mercy with anyone. Children, teens, adults, old people, loving them makes a difference for me, it makes me feel alive. Living knowing you'll die and not knowing when, must me terrible, especially with HIV.

You never know what the reactions are going to be with this illness that it's a monster and you don't know when it's going to attack and kill you. I pray every day for someone to find the cure for this horrible illness. There are nights that my patients call me because they are lonely and scared; others cry like little babies and want me to give them a hug. Others look like they are lost, eyes looking nowhere, they don't understand the reasoning about this illness. Some want me to pray with them, some ask me to tell them a story and some ask me if they disgust me and if I'm not afraid of getting infected. Some of them call me to ask me to give them a hug and tell them I love you. This is very painful for me and it makes my heart sad, I do as much as I can for them but can't do much more other than tell them that I love them, I care for them and console them the nights of pain and suffering.

We wait until they die and then get to put them in a plastic bag. That is something I cannot explain, there is no way to tell you how I feel when something like that happens, it's like the rest of the world doesn't exist, and my heart gets broken in a million pieces. I tell myself, *"I wish I would've done more for them."* Oh God, what a terrible situation but I believe in everything I did for them when they were alive, that's the most important thing. I give them my love and comprehension, especially when they feel so lonely and ignored by the rest of the people. I ask God everyday that goes by to give me more understanding; I want to make sure I give them the best of me. Fight against this illness is not easy; they are like warriors without armor or any other type of protection. They already lost the battle. Lets don't help them make the gravestone before is time; lets make them feel like human beings, not like sick animals.

If Jesus Christ had thought that way he would had left the cross half way and today we would all be lost. If we really care about these people we should do something for them, they don't have the resources or the defenses. They get thrown out of where they live to the streets like they are dogs, they get fired like if they had leper and every time it's a different excuse. The important thing is that we need to change our way of thinking and acting. If we don't we are not going to get too far along. It is very possible we get into their same situation one day and I don't think we would like people to treat us that way. It is easier for us to judge them when we don't see our own defects.

What kind of human beings we are, hypocrites, we don't even know what we want. Shame on us if we think we are exempt of getting AIDS. We should never say never, we can be wrong. What we really need to do is feel more compassion for other people; we never know what can happen to us. I've been very humanitarian since I was a little girl. I always liked to help other people so this job it's very important for me. What counts in here is the ways your parents have teach you. The majority of HIV positive patients are people who never had any love, very lonely since they were children and they had to do things they didn't wanted to do but had to do them anyway in order to survive. This is very sad; they come from very poor communities. No food or money and they have been discriminated against. We don't stop and think about this, we just judge them while we live our lives in good health and with many commodities.

Thousands of children die in NYC everyday because they don't have a place to live. When they need to fight to survive this way it's very hard, that's how they grow up and they are raised. They start stealing in order to get food, and this is only the beginning. As they keep growing they continue to do even worst things, they now need more than food and clothes. Their expenses are higher, they need money for drugs. They don't know how to read or write so they can't get a job so they start to feel abandoned, nobody lends them a hand. They become hard and against everything, nobody wants to get their life complicated with them. That's when the battle starts, stealing and assaulting the first person that goes in their way not worrying about anything.

Society is part to blame; they are always in the middle and being black doesn't help. As they grow up, it gets harder to avoid all of the problems of society. Parents get divorced, the mother is depressed and as you can imagine, who pays for the consequences are the children. They grow up with hate in their hearts; they don't know anything other than suffering. They don't know what it is to be happy or about the happiness that exists in the world, their world it's very dark. They start stealing and killing to support their addiction, which is what sends them to perdition. Then, they realize it is too late. Now they are juvenile delinquents, with no future. Police officers always watching them, forever marked, they start drinking and doing drugs when they are very young. They now had become dangerous and without them even realizing it they end up in jail or the electric chair. They go from one hell to the other and what's worse, becoming HIV positive, and HIV doesn't forgive.

It doesn't matter nationality, skin color or age. It doesn't matter, it affects all of them. There is something very curious that I've learned while working with them. Talking about being discriminated and many other things they all have the same thing in common, HIV positive. There is no color or race for HIV and it's very sad something like this has to happen to make people understand each other. When they start with drugs they only want to test them. When they have all those women they only want to gain experience, nobody wants to get HIV. Now things have change, they can't control anything and HIV has the control.

Since I've been working on this hospital I've had the opportunity to meet many people and its really painful when they tell you all about how much they have suffered having to fight with this illness and all the people that don't even want to see them, and on top of that keep fighting with this illness that has no mercy with them. I pray to God to have mercy with them, they have suffered so much already they don't even have more tears to cry. I know they have a heart of gold, but you have to carve really deep to find it, it is under all that hate and pain. We should not reject them; we should try to understand them. They are human beings like us but they committed a lot of sins, but we have sins too.

Who are we to judge them? We are not better than they are. Before we talk about them we should look at ourselves. It is always easier to see other people mistakes than ours. I give God thanks, he is the one who has inspired me to write this book, and without his help I wouldn't be able to do it. He is love and compassion. He tells me what to do and I obey him because I am His servant. He has thought me to love the ones that nobody loves, to pray for the ones that no one prays for and to understand the ones that nobody understands. These people are in so much need of love and understanding that with only a little bit they are happy. Sometimes the most insignificant things are the most important.

For me, the smallest things are the important ones, those are the ones that make me happy and it is not different for them. It is in the smallest things where the best things are. We sometimes have our eyes so high that we can't see the smallest things and see those are the ones that makes us happy but is always easier to look up and step down. God loves all those small things even thought they look insignificant, nobody can understand it but God. He created many small things we don't give any importance to.

The only things I see at work are suffering and pain. They know they are dying so they don't care anymore. They had told me so many stories it's hard to forget them; they are now part of me.

Other than God, they are my inspiration to write this book so you can understand how they feel and what a blessing is to be healthy and have a family and many other things they are never going to be able to have and we have but don't give it the importance it deserves. I pray to God the cure for AIDS is promptly found and I ask him to help me keep going to keep helping these poor souls. They really need it.

Sometimes I try to put myself on their place but I don't know how to react. God, forgive me if sometimes I'm ungrateful, but I never regret being able to help them, that's why we are here on earth.

14. John's story

It all started one morning I was working at the hospital, it was around 5 a.m. when they took John to his room. He was 27-years-old and was very sick. I talked to him for about half hour, it was almost impossible for him to respond. He was very weak and couldn't breathe. After talking with him I knew he wasn't going to last long so I asked him if he was religious. He told me he believed in God. I told him about something very important I had for him and he told me he was listening. I told him, *"John, you know you are dying and may not make it past tonight."* He agreed, so I asked him if he wanted to accept Jesus Christ like his personal savior and he agreed.

That's how our friendship started. It was time for me to go home; I remember I had a Bible with me so I offered it to him. He got very happy and started reading it immediately and then asked me to tell him more about God. After half hour I went home, my work hours were over but before I left I told him that I would see him again at night.

When I came back, he wasn't there anymore. I asked the nurse what had happened and she told me after I left he got worst and they had to move him ICU. I started praying and asked God not to let him die because he finally found what he had been looking for a long time ago. I wanted to help him read the Bible, show him that even thought he was going to die there was no need to get desperate because God was on his side. Five days went by and I still didn't know anything about him,

I just kept praying. At the sixth day I came back to work and started going through the rooms like every night and what a surprise I had, I felt short of breath when I saw John back in one of the rooms.

I started crying, I couldn't believe it. God had answered my prayers. Thank you God for not taking John with you! Nobody believed how quick John recovered, it was a miracle. John also knew it was a miracle, he was here and now I was going to show him how to read the Bible. We were both really grateful with God, even thou he was still very weak to understand some of the things in the Bible. Days kept passing by and he kept learning from the bible and getting better. He still had a lot to fight with, being HIV positive it's not easy, but like he said, *"this is just another test that I need to get through"*

He wasn't alone now, God was with him. Sometimes we talked about his HIV and how long he had to live but he was very optimistic and wanted to act brave but I knew how he felt inside. I just kept doing everything I could to keep his mind occupied. Other times he will tell me he wished they gave him an injection and kill him once and for all. I asked him how he can be thinking in those things; God is the only one who has that power. He would reply that I didn't understand because I didn't have the virus. If I had the virus I would tell him that I was in God hands and He can cure you when he wants. I wouldn't be afraid, God is with me, He lives with me and knows how I think and how I feel, He is my creator and He would help me move forward.

John asked me if God can help him too and I told him that of course He can. The days that followed John kept reading the Bible and everyday that went by he looked better, he didn't had that look on his face like he was lost and sick like he was when he got to the hospital. I don't know why but he is getting better by the hour, every time I go see him he looks better. God has made a miracle and he knows it. Every time he sees me he gets really happy, he never had a sister in Christ before.

I was talking with him tonight and he told me they are not going to remove any more liquids from his elbows. He had an infection in his elbows that cause them to fill with liquid. They had to extract the liquid with syringes and it is really painful due to the tenderness of the area. Other than that he is getting better fast and quickly. He thanks God for everything He has done for him and so do I. I saw him so sick and now he is getting better so quickly I have to admit this is a miracle. We both know that thanks to God, who always has His hand over us, he is better and I ask Him to keep it this way. This is great proof for John that God is real and He doesn't abandon us. Today we were talking about his life and he promised me he would give me his testimony, he wants others to follow his example. When you have Jesus as your friend you have everything, He has the answers drugs can't give you. Jesus is the answer to everything we are looking for but looks like we can't find it.

Tonight looks like is going to be a calm night and I hope continues that way. I'm pretty tired and with a lot of things in my mind. For example, I'm worried about Gary, he hasn't written to me and that is very strange, he is always very consistent with his letters. On the last letter he sent me he told me he had an infection in one of his fingers. I guess that is the reason he hasn't write to me, usually I receive at least two letters per week. I will continue praying so he gets better and can continue with his letters. I know he feels better when he sends me letters and so do I. I'm so tired my eyes keep shutting down but I can't fall asleep here.

John called me to give me good news. He got me a Bible. I gave him mine when he got here and was really sick. He really didn't have to, I have another one but it makes me feel really happy he feels happy. There are days that the only thing he does is talk about his illness and when he will die and that makes us both depressed. He feels close to God with the Bible, he prays and reads it and that gives him comfort. He also has me to talk; he needs good friends like me.

Being in his situation is good to have somebody who gives you hope, its not easy being alone, especially when you have AIDS and have so much time to think. It is natural he feels that way and we shouldn't make him not think about it, this is something he needs to learn to deal with. John is a very strong person and is doing it well for the most part, he tries to keep his mind occupied so he doesn't think in all the problems he has.

He and I were talking about the HIV. He told me he believed this was a biomedical war or better yet, a bacteriological one because he had heard they found the cure for HIV, but what a surprise after all the people that had died and the ones that are still dying. He also told me he wishes he can get cured because every day that goes by he feels more and more depressed, he is not feeling like himself anymore. It's like he was another person and is not able to think. He asks God every night for the cure. Living like this is worse than suicide. He needs to be strong and continue moving forward, he can't do anything else. The only thing to do is ask God for mercy and strength to continue, we are going to need it, this illness is a very serious thing.

John is very special to me; I really like talking with him. It makes me sad to realize how hard his life has been, violent and agitated; But God's love is so big and He is the only one who can help him with all he has suffered.

John needs a lot of love and comprehension and I will help with all I can but sometimes God is the only one who would be able to help. He is the only one who knows why these things happen. I know that John made a lot of bad things before but he has met God now and when he did those things he was only a child, nobody gave him an opportunity. We should be the ones giving him the opportunity, he deserves it.

He is now a Christian and everything he did before God has already forgiven. Who are we to cast stones at him, when all of us had done things that under Gods eyes are sins? Sins no matter how small or big, are still sins. Maybe one day we would be able to help each other, but now, nobody gives away anything for nothing so the world is getting worse and worse.

The only thing I can say is that John is getting much better since he became a Christian and he is happy to know all his sins have been forgiven. Each day that goes by he has splendor in his face; he looks like a different person. It's a miracle only God could have made. I pray to God to give us the strength to continue, we are going to need it. The way this world is today there is no other thing we can do but pray and ask Him to have mercy with us. I don't believe we alone can continue, it's so complicated that without God we are not going to get anywhere. May God bless all those who have AIDS, only He knows how much they suffer?

15. Angel's story

Today has been a very special day; I had the opportunity to meet Angel. I got to talk to him and he told me about his life, it's pretty interesting, we've been talking about things before he got AIDS. He thinks about his family every day. He was telling me that when his wife was about to give birth he was really worried and wanted to see the baby. After that he started doing drugs. He already had two children that he loved and now they wanted to see if they could have a girl. He remembers when he went to sleep he had his wife on one side and his children on the other. They were happy but things were going bad and one day he was completely immersed.

- *"Sometimes we do things and we don't know why. If somebody would've told me how I was going to end, I would've told them they were lying and making up a tale. Now I see it a little bit clearer but it is too late. I've already lost my family and everything I had because of my drug addiction, and what's worse, I now am HIV positive. I wish I could explain to you how I feel; I need somebody to listen to me and understand me. I know it's hard. The majority of the people don't even want to see me. I pray to God they found a cure fast, if they don't; I really don't know what's going to happen to us. Maybe one day people can understand that we are human beings and we all make mistakes, we all pay for them also."*

I was talking to Angel today and he asked me to tell you that the people who use drugs are not good people. In order to get the drugs they have to steal, kill, and lie. I'm going to tell you what drugs can do to you. After Angel's family abandoned him he felt so lonely he started using drugs more and more frequently. He then started selling them in order to keep his addiction. The drug he was using was really expensive. One day, a friend offered him something new and different. He agreed, he didn't know what was going to happen and when he got into his friends house, he injected Angel with something that hurt. He felt like he was dying, he woke up at the hospital. His so called friend lit up a cigarette while he was unconscious and put in the bed Angel was sleeping. Everything caught on fire.

"When I woke up I had no idea what had happened. The only thing I knew was that my hair was all burned and so were all my clothes. Then it became clear to me what happened. Someone had paid my friend to kill me. I spent a couple months in the hospital recovering from the burns and trying to remember why this happened. When I was discharged I wanted to go home but they told me not to. The building where I used to live was completely destroyed by the fire, my so-called friend cause all of it. All the people who lived there were really upset with me and wanted to kill me. I went there anyway, but if I knew what was waiting for me there, I would've have gone. When I got in front of my house I couldn't believe what my eyes were seeing. I went into what was left of my house and I saw four men that used to live there also. I asked them to forgive me for what I did and for what had happened. It wasn't my fault, I didn't cause the building to get on fire, but they didn't want to listen to me."

"They got really upset and one of them hit me in the head leaving me unconscious. They took all my clothes and naked, they started hitting me with wood sticks, to kick me all over my body and to punch me. When they were done I looked like hamburger meat. They hit me until they got tired of it. They had me tied up all day. All of the sudden I heard a dog barking. A man that heard the dog barking saw me there and called an ambulance and they took me back to the hospital. For six months I was in there, almost died. All I did in that time was to think of what I was going to do when I got out of there. Days were so long it felt like it was never going to end.

While there all I thought was how to solve everything when discharged. I really didn't know why my friend betrayed me and I didn't know who sent him to kill me."

"I had no idea what was going on and when the time came to leave the hospital I still couldn't believe it, it was like a dream. I thought to myself, I'm going to go find the person who did this to me. I knew it wasn't going to be easy but I had to try. So I went to find the first one, you have to start somewhere, right? While looking I found my "friend" and I gave him such a beating for everything he made me suffered and for trying to kill me. After that I went to look for the second one but it was a little harder, I couldn't get a way to find him, it was like he disappeared from earth. But the day came when I found him and I give him a beating that he will remember me for forever. I told him that if he didn't give me the name of the other two guys it was going to be very hard for his family to recognize him. He refused to talk so I almost broke his arm until he finally talked. I asked him for the addresses and I warned him to do it or else. He told me he didn't know the addresses, only that they were in Puerto Rico."

"I went to Puerto Rico and found one of them before looking through the whole island. We had a long conversation and he gave me the address for the last one. Before I left, I gave him a beating so he could remember me all his life. I sent him to the hospital for six months, the same time I spent at the hospital too. All I did all this time was think about my family. I wanted to die, I had so many things to do I didn't wanted to leave half done. I had to finish what I've already started. I couldn't forget about all what happened. I kept looking. Only God knew where he was. Sooner or later he had to appear so I kept looking. I knew he was close to me, I just needed to wait. At the same time my brother learned that somebody else was looking for me to kill me."

"My brother decided to help me look for the person who was supposed to kill me and when he found it my brother convince him not to do it. He promised my brother he would not hurt me. All I wanted to know is who paid him to kill me. He just told me that there were many people involved in all this. I kept looking for the forth guy but he was much smarter than

the last three so it was getting harder for me to find him. I went to all his friends' houses with no luck. One day he came back from Puerto Rico and went straight to the Bronx. I kept looking for him in Puerto Rico without knowing he was back in the Bronx. When I thought I'd lost him I found one of his friends and he told me the other guy was in NYC already. I came back to the city and started looking for him again."

"My brother and his friends knew where he was hiding and they told me. I asked them to come get him with me and not let him escape. I didn't want them to get involved; I wanted to be the one who confronted him. They all agreed so we went straight to where he lived. When he saw me, he started running but my brother's friends didn't let him go. I confronted him and asked him why he did the things he did to me, I never did anything bad to him before. He agreed with me but told me that what happened with the fire was my fault. I told him that it wasn't my fault, that other crazy guy is the one who burned the building. He didn't have any right to do what he did with me. It was my turn now. "Let me explain to you how things work here."

"So I gave him such a beating that he was in the hospital for six months. I had already finished with the battle and was ready to start all over again. I didn't want to think about anything, I've lost everything. I started going woman after woman and living large. I'm not going to tell you how I got the money, that is nobody's business, but I'll tell you that I needed $300.00 a day to support my vices and there was no way I could've earn that money working on a regular job. Gradually, I started declining to the point I got sick. I tried to commit suicide a couple of times with no luck, God didn't want me dead. Now I understand why, he wants my testimony for everybody to know that if you do things the wrong way you'll end wrong and that He is in control of everything. He is above it all."

"Josefina, I'm really scared. I don't know what's coming next, and all I can say is that I give God thanks for sending you my way. You are a solace for me and I want you to know that I appreciate every minute you spend here with me listening. You are a very special person and I know God is the one who sent you to help me while I live through this agony. But I don't

despair, if I die, I know I'm going to heaven praise the Lord. Many times I realize that if someone had told me what drugs do to you I wouldn't be where I am today. What's done is done. We can't go backwards. Since we had made these mistakes out of ignorance we don't want you to make our same mistakes. This is why I'm helping Josefina, so she can tell us about all these things and many more. If you ever read this book I urge you to understand that life is not how they picture it in TV. Drugs would make you do things that you can't imagine. And this I tell you very seriously. I don't want any of you to end up like me, young and with no future. A whole life ahead of me and I will not be able to enjoy it. This is very painful to me, I know life is not easy but drugs are not the answer to your problems. Respect your bodies, this is what God has given to you and you should treat it like a gardener treats his garden. Jail is no place for anyone. There are only two places you are going to end up at, jail or the cemetery. Quite frankly, I don't know which one is worse. If you die, you are dead but being dead alive is a horrible thing."

"Maybe one day God would give us the opportunity to speak with him in person so you can see that what I'm telling you are not lies. This is not a dream, you need to wake up, face the reality and walk to the light because you are not going to find anything in the darkness. When I thought I was lost I saw a tunnel with a light inside. I followed the light just to see where it could take me and I found the answer to what I was looking for. I found the truth, the path and the light that was going to guide me for the rest of my life. That answer is Jesus Christ. I feel much better now in his hands, I know I'm free of any dangers. I urge you to follow the light, where there is light there can't be darkness, in the darkness you can trip and hurt yourself."

"Sometimes I feel lonely and I cry like a baby and wish I could go back and start over, but when you take a step like the one I took, nothing can take you back and nobody would give you back all you lost."

As you can see, Angel doesn't have any more hope than one thing and that thing is Jesus. I'm going to tell you something about Angel that you don't know. He has two tubes inserted in his side that go directly to his lung. That is one surgery, plus another three tubes in his chest.

This is how they can inject him antibiotics and how they draw blood out of him for testing. He is HIV positive and his veins are no longer good and this is the only way they can draw blood out of him. He is gradually consuming himself. He gets skinnier every day but with a wonderful sense of humor. He is a great guy.

If you think this is life, every time he takes his medication he throws up. He has very high fevers and I want you to imagine how much he suffers and how much makes me suffer seeing him like this and not being able to do anything for him. This is very sad for me but I need to be strong and keep going. Sometimes he calls me and asks me things that I don't really know how to answer him. For example, why he can't get married and have sex, and why he can't have children because of AIDS. Sometimes he tells me: *"Maybe I'll find a girl that has AIDS too and we can start a new life."*

I just laugh with him. He can be very funny and will try to cheer me up but I am crying inside. I see him suffer so much and so lonely. The only thing I can do for him is encourage him and tell him he can't think like that but if he really needs a wife is not a bad idea. He has told me that he can never *"deceive a woman who is healthy but if I go out with an HIV positive girl that is not a problem."* I told him that is not a bad idea, I don't know if he tells me that to make me feel better or he is serious about it. Maybe I will never know, I don't think he wants to hurt me or see me suffer. You need to understand that the sufferings of these people are so big that the Pacific Ocean is small compared to it. I always ask God to give them a short life.

There is a lot going on tonight at the hospital. It's like everybody in the hospital got in accordance and all the patients are restless. I have met a very interesting character today. He's a very nice and happy old man that call me a couple of times and when I went to see what he needed all he wanted was attention like a young child. He told me that he went to war and had won a gold medal for saving his regiment. He got recognized and today he is a hero. Very pleasant person, he is Italian. I ask him what was wrong with him and he told me that he was very lonely and needed to talk to somebody. I asked him what he wanted to talk about and he told me to shave him because he felt dirty. All of the sudden a nurse called me to go help her with one of our patients who were very sick.

The night progressed with work every five minutes. It was like all the patients got in accordance to feel bad. It was unbelievable. I'm not afraid of working, especially when I know they need me. I've been in around so many times tonight I don't even know where to put my feet. I wish I could rest but I can't. The patients ask me for water, food, sodas, others are in a total depression and I have to talk to them so they get better self esteem. The first thing they think is on suicide and we can't let that happen. I'm happy to be here, close to them, because I know they need me and I'm here to help. This makes me feel good even though I'm tired.

Everything I do, I do correctly and I'm happy to know that they think this way. There is no shame in knowing somebody needs you, to the contrary, it is an honor for me to help them in whatever they need. We should be happy we can help somebody. I ask God to give me the strength to keep going until the end and that everything I do is for his glory. He is the one who has given us our life and he owns it. Sometimes I ask myself what would happen if there were more people like me and I think everything would be much better, don't you think?

It is hard; when they are dying you don't know what to do or what to think. Only that your heart hurts and we can't do anything. We can't change the route that has already being traced. The only thing we can do its help each other the best way we can, we never know what destiny life has for us. We need to do the things that are right and without complaints even thou this can seem harder. Nobody said we were perfect, right? At least we can do what's right.

16. Gary's story

I received a letter from Gary today. He tells me he is very depressed and not doing well. The medicines that the doctor gave him had given him anemia, he's destroyed and bored. He asked me how long can he stay like that and I don't know what to tell him. Truth is he is so depressed, I don't know how he feels. Thinking about how little life you have ahead of you is not very funny, especially for him. I prayed to God to give him strength because I don't know what to tell him. It makes me feel so bad to think I can give him strength when I'm so sad too, I don't know what to tell him. Sometimes I ran out of words, is not easy to give encouragement when you are also depressed. Sometimes I feel like they feel, trapped in a box with no escape. I wish I could do miracles but is not easy to see them this way.

17. Angel, continued

Today I was talking with Angel. We were talking about when his time comes to go. He told me, *"Very soon, the doctors told me I was much better but I'm so sad that I have to go. I will miss you so much. I've asked God to give me a short life."* I told him that he didn't have to worry, everything is going to be alright and thank God and he got happier.

There are times in life that we do things that we should've not done. When you start regretting it, it's just too late for that. Angel, I want you to know that as a sister in Jesus Christ, I love you and so does my family. We are never going to abandon you. I pray to God to give me the strength to finish my book. It is not easy to write about these people without feeling pain inside me.

Angel asked me a question and I started shaking because I didn't know what to expect from him. *"Josefina, I'm scared, I don't know what is going to happen with me, you have more experience than me. You've seen the people in here everyday, you know how much we suffer and how little life we have left"* and I responded."

"Angel, I wish I could do something else for you, but you know I don't have magic powers. What I do have is an incredible faith in God and I know he is going to help you. He has already forgiven you for everything you did. You need to stay positive; if you are negative you are going to be done before you even start. The only other thing I can tell you is that if there is God, there is hope and He is the one who has all the answers.

Leave everything in His hands. Angel, I know it is very difficult to be in your situation but we can't really do much more. I know that some day not far from today God is going to open the doors for all those who are HIV positive. Be patient, He knows what he is doing and I never lose hope. I sure hope God listens to my prayers; we are going to need them. Everyday that goes by there are more people with AIDS. It's like a never ending story. Maybe one day soon we would be able to see science achievements to find a cure. We need to be patient, even when we know they are millions dying. I understand you are lonely, and I can share that with you but you have to think of your reality, what's already been done and you and I can't change even in a thousand years".

Sometimes when I'm taking a break at work I start thinking and a million things go through my mind. I'm fully exposed to have one infected syringe pinch my skin. What's going to happen to me next? I get goose bumps just thinking about getting HIV. Everything in life has a price that we would need to pay one way or the other.

18. Christopher's story

Tonight is a very quiet night. I'm done with taking the temperatures of the patients; I have collected the dirty clothes from the rooms and replaced them with clean ones. There are the same things every night. We have a patient here that is HIV positive and it really sick. His whole family came to visit him today.

It is so painful and inexplicable to see Christopher's whole family seeing him suffer like that and not be able to do anything. He is dying and all he is able to say tonight is that he wants to be dead. I spent some time talking with his mom, his brothers and other relatives and I can't believe how much a little bit of love and understanding can do. They don't know what to do; they are just waiting for him to be done with his agony. It is now 3:30 am and everything is still calm besides a couple of patients that had called me to get them water or to talk to me.

Today I'm confused; it really affects me, especially because Christopher is one of my favorites. I have many and very special memories and moments with him, I have had enough time to get to know him well. And now that he is about to die I feel like some part of me is dying too. I can't really do anything for him, just console him and pray to God not to let him suffer more. Sometimes I would get into his room, just to check how he was doing, because we expected him to die at any moment now. I was really nervous and had a very bad stomach ache.

It is not easy to hide your emotions, especially when you are in constant contact with them all the time. Maybe one day I'll be able to take away this pain I feel inside me that feels like its eating me like a cancer. I wish somebody can be on my place; it is not easy and can get very depressing. I thank God every day, He is the one that gives me the strength to keep fighting and I praise Him every day. I know that I wouldn't be able to do it all by myself. Every single day I see the relatives of the sick patients, I share the good moments and the bad moments. What they don't know is that when they leave, the patients are fragile like little children and they find shelter on me. They ask me to just listen to them, to answer questions about why they have to die. The only thing I can do is listen to them, give them advice and talk to them about God.

Sometimes they feel so isolated from everybody that they ask me to hug them and to hold their hand. They ask me why I'm not afraid of getting HIV and while I write this, Christopher is dying. The only thing I can remember is that this past Christmas I got my children to the hospital so they can meet him because he wanted to meet them. I remember he was so happy; my children were really good with him.

The patients act really strong in front of their families. They don't want their families to see them cry or think they are weak. It shouldn't be like that. Is in these moments were they need their families the most. They can hide it very well and suffer when they are all by themselves. Truth is, nobody knows how it feels; they are the ones who are dying. If we traded places, I don't know how we would act or what we would do in that situation. It is not easy to know you are dying and you can't do anything. It a constant battle with an enemy you can defeat. They, however, keep fighting. If they don't fight for the days they have left their illness would defeat them in just a couple days. I only speak from what they tell me and from what I see. I give them strength, but when I'm alone or writing for my book I get to think that I wish they were more people like me, understanding and affectionate, they really need people like that. They are confused and don't know how to get out, how to escape.

It's been five minutes since Christopher died. This is terrible; I feel like I have a fireball in my stomach it hurts me so much. At least he is not suffering anymore. Another victory for HIV, another victim he has gained. When I went to his room I found him so rigid and pale that I was paralyzed when I saw him. Then, his mother came out of the room crying and followed by his brother. It was all really depressing. His mother saw me and came hug me and said only one thing to me, *"Thank you Lord that he is not going to suffer anymore."*

She calmed down with my hug and we didn't say anything else to each other. We didn't need any other words to understand us. His journey through hell was over, all the relatives are gone and now we have to clean him, put tags on his feet, tie his arms and legs and gag his mouth so it doesn't opens. While I'm doing this all I think is that half hour ago he still had his eyes open. I was thinking that now he doesn't have anything to worry about, he would not have any more accidents in his bed, or any of the other things that bother him so much. So many things go through my mind. One thing I can't forget is how he kept saying that he wanted to die. All this going through my mind while I'm placing his body inside the plastic bag.

We are nothing. Sometimes we think we are so big and powerful; if only we knew what was going to happen to all of us at the end, we would be more humble and benevolent. We would appreciate more all those moments that we go through in our life. Every moment we have of life is precious and we should use it for good things and to better understand others. We just now finished preparing the body. It is now ready to take out of here. I'm done for today. It is time for me to go home, send my children to school and try to rest if I can.

Today I went out and got the newspaper to find out when it's Christopher's funeral. I was very surprised with what I found. I found the day of the funeral but I also found something else that hurt me even more. His family posted that he died at the San Pedro Hospital and that he died of cancer. The truth is that he died at Albany Medical and he died of AIDS. I don't understand why so many lies. I can't understand why they have to be ashamed to tell that his son died of AIDS. This is what I call ignorance. This is one of the reasons I work with them. I'm not ashamed of them, they are human beings like you and I. I feel respect for them and I have enough love to take care of them and to tell them they are not alone. God is with them and so am I. We need to help them understand they are human beings and even thou they made a mistake, like Jesus said when they were going to stone Mary Magdalene "He who is without sin should cast the first stone". It is easy for us to see other people's sins but not ours. Who are we to judge others?

19. Gary, continued

I received a letter from Gary today. He tells me he feels much better and he misses us. Gary it's a very special case. He has the need to feel he has friends and that's why he always writes to me. He tells me how are things going and how his AIDS progresses. He doesn't know when he is going to die, but he knows he has a dead sentence like many others that have his illness.

There's so much medical testing they go through and so many medicines they take and for what? They each have their days counted. Sooner or later, they all end up at jail and with AIDS. This is very serious, they are human beings and we need to help them make their days easier.

I think that, instead of hiding that somebody has died of AIDS, we should tell everybody how many people die from AIDS every day. We all care more about what our friends are going to say if they find out somebody in our family died of AIDS. What kind of world we live in that we are ashamed of our own blood? I pray to God to give me the strength to keep helping those who need me, all those who need moral and spiritual support and help them die in peace and in God's grace. Amen.

Tonight's a very quiet night and all the patients are sleeping. I feel very lonely today. I have nobody to talk to. Angel is gone and so are other patients. I feel a terrible emptiness today, like my heart wants to get out of its place.

I really appreciate them and this is what happens when you get to be their friend and then they go away. I feel like something has died inside me. I will now have to start over, all my patients are gone. I know more will come, but it's never going to be the same. The only thing I can do is wait to see if any of them would remember me and write me letters. It's painful and I pray to God to give me the strength to continue, I don't think I can do it alone. So many dead patients in so little time, I can't believe it. I would've never thought I would need to gag so many mouths of the patients who die here; somebody has to do the dirty work. You just get used to it; it's like a bad dream. Everyone that dies in here is so young. I feel so sad, but this is my job and I have to do it. I pray to God to give me strength to help me help them because they really need it.

Maybe one day I'll be able to understand this loneliness inside me. I know that the ones that have left are going to miss me. I took care of them with all my heart and did everything I could for them. Today is a very sad day, I know that sooner or later they will come back here and that makes me happy and at the same time sad. Usually when they come back it is for their last stop. It feels like they are coming to say goodbye. I stay with them all through the process and it is not fun at all. The fact that they die in your hands is not pleasant even thou I take care of them with all I can and it's my pleasure. Sometimes the hospital assigns me to other departments and I spend the night with different patients. This gives me the opportunity to rest and to think about other things. It is not good to be thinking about them all the time; you will end up sick too. I think of them constantly, I live with them and share their feelings. Many times I would like to go to sleep and don't think about it. I even have dreams about them. It is like I am a Vietnam War Veteran. It is worse than a nightmare or a horror movie that is never going to end. Unfortunately, they play with the worst cards and are destined to lose.

20. Jose

I was talking today to José. He was telling me how upset he is. Doctors would not tell him his tests results and he is very worried. They had put a Hickman is his body. A Hickman is a machine they put in your chest to draw blood so they don't have to pinch your veins. His veins don't work anymore. He was telling me that he is HIV positive and that when he got to the hospital he had to sign paperwork giving the doctors consent to treat him. The doctors can not treat him without his consent.

He told the doctor that he couldn't see very well from one eye and the doctor gave him some eye drops for the irritation. He told the doctor that he *"believed that is something more serious than an irritation because I can see at all and it keeps getting worst. The doctor told me not to worry, that it was nothing."*

"As the days went by, I felt worst and worst. Lab after lab, one thing after the other and I had no idea what was going on. Some days with high fevers, other days normal and others that I thought I wasn't going to make it. Always a different medication, many times with very violent results. I would throw up everything. Food here is terrible, I wish I didn't have to take the medicines, they are driving me crazy. Sometimes I don't even know who I am, totally confused. Because of the doctor not listening to me, I have lost total vision in one eye, if they would have listen to me maybe today I would've been able to see again. Now it's going to the other eye. It is an

infection and the treatment I was going through had to be stopped due to the fact that it has eliminated all my white blood cells and I have no immune defense. I am extremely worried; I don't know what to do. Sometimes I wish I die, but I guess I'll die when it's my turn to."

"I asked the doctor when he was going to give me the results of my tests. I wanted to know how things were going. I told him that I had it with all the medication. He told me that he didn't know when I would have the results. This made me very mad and I told him, "Of course it's not important to you. We are just rats for your medical experiments."

The doctor got really upset and told me, 'When you got in here you signed a paper giving us permission to give you drugs and now that we are doing it you are complaining. What do you want us to do with you?" I told him, "I wish you would be a little more humanitarian with me. This is very painful to us; you are so used to dealing with patients. Do you think we are animals? I know you do not perform miracles and that you are not geniuses but can you please have a little compassion with us? You didn't listen to me before and now I'm going blind and that is not funny. I already know what I'm going to do, I can't expect anything. I know I'm dying. All of you are so used to seeing people dying that you don't feel any compassion anymore. I don't know where we are going with all this; I hope that this ends quickly. I'm not sure how much time I can resists in here. I'm slowly declaiming and it is a shame, I don't want to die. There is nothing I can do. I know sooner or later I'm going to die.""

"Sometimes when I'm by myself I think of being able to go back and start all over again. I want to get so many things I haven't got and do so many things I haven't done. The only thing I can do is daydream. Oh good heavens! What was I thinking when I got into this mess? It's too late to regret anything. All I can do is pray to God that he can help me; I know I can't do it by myself. My dad was right. He once told me: "Doctors are human beings that also make mistakes, but you have to put all your faith in God. He is the one that makes miracles and he is the one that can take all you problems away. Keep your head up and you will see the light you need to follow."

"Josefina, I don't think they are going to find the AIDS cure. I think this is all a fraud and I'll tell you why I think that way. Do you remember when they were talking about killing African Americans? And they were doing chemical experiments to take them out of the way? Then we heard for the first time, around 1972 if I'm not mistaken, that the first case of AIDS came from Africa and that it was a virus that monkeys carried, I don't get it. If that's true, why they don't stop it? I think the government has done this to get rid of minorities. I find it absurd to eliminate people this way. Can you think of a better way of taking people out of the way? If knew it, I wouldn't be there today. But it can be true, I have no doubts. What a way to take people out of the way. What do you think of HIV? Do you think they are going to find a cure? Or do you think this is the end for the people with AIDS? I really don't want to end my life this way. I'm young, I'm only 32. I have all my life ahead of me. It is so sad that you have to lie to everybody. You have to tell them that you are sick but can't tell them you have AIDS. They all go running away when you tell them. You feel abandoned, sad and lonely. You have to lie in order to keep living. All this is very depressing. I don't know what's best, dying today or keep fighting for the little life I have ahead of me. I really don't know what to do, this is worst than living in hell."

"I believe you José. I want you to answer a couple of questions for the book that I'm writing. How do you really feel?"

"First of all, I feel very alone and I feel a deep emptiness inside me. I wish I could get married and have children like everybody else but I can't have sex with anybody because of the HIV or have children, they will be born with HIV too. That I couldn't forgive myself. This is why I'm telling you that I don't know what to do. I would like to have a house and make my family happy. Josefina, I pray to God that if anybody reads your book they understand how much affection we need. We don't have anybody, for me everything is lost. But there are a lot of people with HIV and they can help them feel better by showing compassion to them. I'm sitting here in my bed waiting for my final moment to come. It seems so far away and it is so painful. I am always crying or worried, I don't know how to respond

to was happening to me. Sometimes I think this is all a bad dream, then I wake up and face reality and everything around me is real. I start thinking everything is going to end soon. I just ask that anybody that reads this book gets moved and helps somebody with AIDS. It is such a shame that for a mistake or an error everybody turns their back on us. Nobody is perfect; we all make mistakes and have sins. Every day I have a different complication with my illness; it's a never ending story. I pray to God I have short life, I don't think I'll be able to resists this for a long period of time. Nobody knows what it is to be like this, just waiting to die. This is something I don't wish even to my worst enemy. Nobody knows what it is to be counting the hours, the minutes, the seconds fly by like they are birds of fire. Every time they approach me they burn more and more. I don't know what else to tell you just that it is very lonely to be like this. I pray to God that even that I know I'm going to die soon; they can find the cure for AIDS."

"This is such a painful and lonely illness. Nobody knows the suffering we have inside us. It's so dark and cold, I get so afraid and mellow that I don't know what to do and I can't control myself. I don't want my family to know that I am HIV positive. This is why I'm here and not at my house, so they don't see me suffer. I love my family and I don't want them to suffer for something I did. I feel so lonely; I don't have anybody to talk other than you. You understand me and know I don't want to make my family suffer. It's sad but I don't want anybody to laugh at my family because I have AIDS. I would never be able to forgive myself."

"My family is very important to me and I could've not resist people rejecting my family because of my illness. So, as you can see this is the way my life is, waiting for my turn. I really hope is quick and fast. I had it with all the suffering and I think I have already paid my dues. Don't you think? I think you are right when you tell me not to get desperate and if I have faith there is hope even when we don't understand why. Of course, I understand and I give God thanks that he sent you to keep me company so I don't feel lonely. Your company gives me comfort. Your jokes make me happy and when you say the beautiful things you say I feel so much better. I know there are worst things in life. Thank you God for all your blessings *and I ask you to forgive me and to bless me. Amen. I'm here waiting for the end to come.*

The most important part of the hospital is C4. This is where we have the patients that have AIDS. They are very special patients and nobody wants them in the other areas of the hospital. This is very strange to me. Instead of looking at the illness, we should look at the fact that they are human beings. We forget that we can also get AIDS. It doesn't have to come from them, it can come from anywhere else, and it all depends on what we have done before. What can we do, life is like a merry-go-round - when it's your turn, and it's your turn.

Yesterday, while I was off, one of my patients died. They were doing a liver test on him. This was the third one in the last two months and his body couldn't resist. He died on the surgery table. Life goes on like nothing happened. Human life doesn't have any value here. All these experiments are horrible and it looks like it's never going to end. I've never thought I would see the things I see here. With every day that goes by, I have more faith in God.

In here you can trust no one, even the doctors. The one who doesn't take your blood out wants to take your money. You tell me what kind of life is this. I'm not sure where we are going or where we are going to end.

Gary's friend

Tonight it's been a night full of surprises. I've met a friend of Gary's. I spend a lot of time talking to him and he told me he reads the Bible and all his sisters are Christians. I ask him when he was going to convert and he told me that he doesn't know how. I told him that this was no coincidence; God sent him my way from jail to have him talk to me about becoming a Christian. God has a way to do things, and when He does, things go very well. When we try to do things by ourselves, we ruin everything. He told me what happened to him; he was being treated but didn't felt better. He told the correctional officer, but he didn't listen and now he was in a lot of pain. Doctors kept visiting him. Running lab test after lab test.

Then he was transferred to the Jail Hospital. When he arrived, they performed so many tests on him. He was scared and didn't know what was going on. He now had three bumps in the left side of his neck and he doesn't know what they were going to do to him. But God is always by our side.

21. John's story

John is a patient with HIV and he is going to tell us his testimony. God, give him the strength to do it. He feels very sick.

It all started when they took him to the correctional hospital and they put him on the surgery table with very little anesthesia. He was afraid what he was very ill. The doctors cut a small incision in his neck. He asked them what they were doing and the doctors told him that he didn't need to worry; they were going to get it all done at once. The two doctors looked more like butchers.

One put his hand on John's neck and removed a bump then did the same thing two more times. When they started to pull, I screamed at them, *"Please don't pull anymore, it really hurts!"*

"The doctors told me to stop screaming at them, that I was crazy because I wasn't in pain at all because of the anesthesia. I told them that I wished that was true, I could really feel all they were doing to me. I asked for something for my pain and they told me to shut up or they were going to hurt me even more. I started screaming like a crazy person to the point that the security guards came to me and asked me what was wrong. I told them the doctors were hurting me and I didn't have enough anesthesia and they didn't care to give me something more for the pain. The security guards told the doctors they didn't have any right to treat people like that."

"Then, they decided to stop working on me and leave the procedure half way done. The security guards told the doctors it was enough already

and what they were doing was butchering me. They took me to jail again. I really hope they treat other people better, what they were doing to me was really painful. When they were taking out the third lump, it felt like they were taking my entire chest out, lungs and everything. I felt like my heart was getting moved out of place. I've never experience something as painful as that. I prayed to God to take me out of that situation. I was about to start throwing punches to everybody. What they were doing with me was not of human character. They don't care; they are not the ones in pain. It is very sad there are so many doctors in this world lacking compassion. But, because I'm a prisoner they assume I have to pay for what I have done before. Still, that is not the right way. They are not entitled to make me suffer like that. The pain was unbelievable. It felt like they were cutting my neck little by little, like I was dying. When I got to the correctional hospital they took care of me the best way they could. I stayed there for two months."

"After that, the other side of my neck started bothering me but doctors couldn't find what was wrong with me, so they sent me back to jail. After a couple days I felt a lump under in my underarm. They told me not to worry about it, that it was just some minor inflammation. I knew that it wasn't over yet. The three lumps in my neck came back and the doctors almost killed me, they told me they were taking me to the Albany Hospital because in there they were going to treat me better and they had more experience with cases like mine."

"When I arrived at the Albany Hospital everybody treated me different. That's how I met Josefina. I told her everything that happened to me and she told me she was writing a book. I volunteered myself and asked her if she had space for one more testimony in her book. She said yes. That same night Josefina talked to me about Jesus Christ and explained to me He was the only one that could help me because I was HIV positive. The pain I had was unbearable but I continued to listen to what she had to say about Jesus Christ. She asked me where I wanted to go when I died, Heaven or Hell. I told her I wanted to go to Heaven because I already had enough Hell here on Earth."

"She introduced me to Jesus. That same night I accepted Jesus Christ in my heart and I'm really happy about it. I know if something happens to me I'm going to Heaven, I have Jesus Christ in my heart."

"I'm no longer alone. I'm waiting to have another surgery. I believe is going to be on my right side today. The lump I have is getting bigger and bigger so I'm praying to God. I want to thank Him for being so good to me and I want to tell everybody what Jesus Christ has done for me. When He does something for us we should share it with everybody else. He does a lot of miracles every day. Now I have eternal life, something I didn't have before. I thank Him every day and praise Him. Amen".

After three days of speaking with John they took him to surgery. That day was my day off but John told me his wife was going to go see him at the hospital. She wanted to be with him after surgery. I went home, and five hours later I went back to the hospital to find out how where things going but he was still waiting for the surgery and his wife was there with him. I introduced myself and stayed with her and invited her to the cafeteria to have some coffee and keep her busy.

She was very worried about her husband. She is the sweetest person I've ever met. Friendly and humble. She was taking it all very well, getting a little nervous from time to time. We didn't know how things were going on the surgery table. She was also a Christian and she had a faith in God to help his husband get out of it. When the time came that I had to go I gave her my phone number and told her if she needed something to call me.

Next day when I came back to work, he was in bed and in a lot of pain. It has been two days since he had surgery and had a really high fever. Days passed by and he looked like he was feeling better. We talked about the stupid things we do in life and how pricey they can be. There is nothing like having good friends. A few days later, he looked like he was getting better, except his fever would make him feel like he was dying. He looked like he was getting better, with some good days and some bad days.

What can we do? Such is life. He got much better with time and it was incredible the way he got better from one day to the other. God is the only one responsible for this miracle. Feeling good from one day to the other, the doctors couldn't explain how that happened. They couldn't believe it.

But like I said, having Jesus on our side makes everything go our way, that is of course if we behave the way Jesus want us to behave. We need to give God thanks every day. Without him I'm not sure where we would be. We are here because he has placed us here for some reason. He uses his own logic even thou we can't always understand why. We should leave God's things alone; He is the only one who knows how everything works.

22. James' story

I met James a long time ago. The first time I saw him he was escorted by the police and they chained him to his bed by his hands and feet. They were treating him like a criminal. He was very sick and very skinny. They then told me he had suffered from something very similar to an epileptic attack, and the police officers had found him on the streets. After two days they took the handcuffs away and he looked like he was doing better.

He spent a lot of time in the hospital and I asked him if he knew Jesus Christ. He told me he was a Christian. I continued seeing him every day until he got better and they released him from the hospital. He didn't have any friends and the ones he had were all involved with drugs. What I would like to tell you about is how he got to be HIV positive.

When he was a little boy his parents sent him to one of those places you put children when you don't want them. A place where you abandon children and they receive no love whatsoever or learn how to give love. They grow up like little cubs, not knowing how they are going to get out of there without hurting themselves. He told me the only things he learned in there was how to fight, how to steal and other things- all of them bad and nothing good. He had to survive that entire calamity or he was going to die.

He grew up without love and that was really sad. He didn't know how to express affection. That must have been very sad for him, to have a life like that. When you are a child you need to feel the love and the affection from your parents. He grew up and kept doing whatever he needed to do to survive. His life was very difficult and instead of getting better he was getting worst. His friends where taking him to the wrong path of life. They introduced him to drugs. They helped each other, like a family, since they were the only family they knew. It didn't matter what they did, nobody cared about all those children at the place they were at.

He told me, with tears in his eyes, that he didn't have anybody. He grew up without love, with no one to say "I love you" or to give a hug to. That really breaks my heart. I have three children I don't want anything like that to happen to them. As years went by, he grew up and kept on being alone. The only thing he knew how to do was stealing and to do whatever he needed to do to survive. It wasn't easy to find the money to maintain his vices and everything was very expensive. Stealing was easy money and the only way to get things. He had to move forward at any cost. He smoked so many drugs and injected so many others that today he is HIV positive.

It is very sad, he tells me he is dying and he hasn't had the opportunity to meet somebody that can make him happy.

But he did found the answer to his sufferings, he found Jesus Christ and He loves him and takes care of him. He also found my family who also loves him and takes care of him. Now he is happy even that he knows he'll die soon. He found the answer to what he was looking for so long. Now, all he has to do is wait until is his time to die.

Now he is never alone, he has Jesus Christ. He reads the Bible every day and that gives him the strength to continue. God helps him every day to continue the fight with his illness.

Sometimes, when I have a day off, I go to see him at the hospital and talk to him. He is very lonely and needs to talk to somebody. He doesn't have anyone. Today, when I went back to work, I stopped to see him, but he wasn't there. They told me he was gone. I was very surprised because the day before I went and talked to him and he told me he would be at the hospital for some time. I may never see him again. Now I have to be patient and wait.

Every day that goes by, I feel different. I wish I had the money to help them. To have a place where I can take care of all the ones who don't have a place to go. It's very painful to see them so sad. The money the government gives to them is not enough to have something to eat. I pray to God to give me strength to keep going. He is the one who gives me power to keep going as is very hard to see them like that and not being able to do anything for them. Only God knows how much I would like to do for them. With God's help and my book I may be able to afford a place where I can take care of them.

Right now I don't have the money but I do have the will to make it happen someday since this is America. Some of them don't have anything. It's very hard for me; you get depressed even if you don't want to. You don't know what to do. It's like having your hands and feet tied. I put everything in God's hands. He is the one guiding me.

Sometimes I think that if we would stop for 10 minutes and look back we would see the people in need but we are always in such a hurry we don't have time to help our neighbors. Try to help the ones that need you. I believe that would make us more human and happier. When I feel down, I go outside to my terrace and look at the birds and how they live and survive. They look so happy! They have food they share with each other or sometimes they fight for it and that reminds me of people, when they have what they need they don't remember the one that has nothing. But when they don't have anything they start to moan like little children. I believe we need to give everybody an opportunity. God gives us so much and forgives us so many others things. It is a shame since we are here only a short period of time and in that time we should help each other more.

Especially when I'm here at work, I realized we are here one day and can be completely gone the other. I feel very good helping my patients and helping everyone that needs me. That is love, being able to love somebody you hardly know. I think what some people need is learn to love his neighbor like they love themselves. Every time I pray I ask

God to give me more of that love to share it with everyone that gets in my path. The only way we can win this battle is by loving each other. It looks like it would be hard to love someone you don't know but if you have Jesus Christ in your heart it's really easy.

The only thing you have to do is ask Him to give you some of His love; He is a millionaire in love. All you have to do is think if he didn't have that love, he would've not let the crucifixion to happen. His life wasn't easy; he left all his treasures at heaven to come suffer for us. He was poor; He didn't have a house or anything to wear other than what he was wearing. All He did He did it for love to us. The kind of love only He knows to offer. And because he loved us so much he paid with his life and then came to life again to give us the opportunity to understand that with love everything is possible.

There is not a lot of His love here on Earth and that's why we have so many problems in this world. People distinguish each other on what color their skin is and how much they know. Love doesn't have a color or a flavor, it's pure.

For example, I'm from Spain with dark skin. I'm not considered white or black, but a lot of white people look at me and they rude comments. Some black people do the same thing; they look at me like I'm something weird and they don't know where I came from.

Love doesn't have any color. For God we are all the same. If we knew how to love we wouldn't see any difference in color. This is why we need to follow Jesus Christ's steps. This way it would be easier for us to love each other. If we follow his steps, He would give us all the love we need to share with the people that need it most. He is like a never-ending fountain of love. He has given us eternal life and never-ending love. This is why I want to follow my master's steps because he loves everyone the same. Color and nationality don't matter. When you have love in your heart, you don't look for defects in another person. I sometimes feel bad when people treat me badly due to my skin color.

All I think is that Jesus Christ doesn't care I have dark skin. Its better this way, instead of going to the beach to tan, I go to church instead to share with my brothers and sisters from church. My King, my Master and my Savior. I think the devil has already way too many souls in hell, lets win the fight. Get yourself full of love and start offering it to anybody that needs it. Many people commit suicide due to lack of love. No one has stop for a second and look back and think they needed love; because they didn't have love they commit suicide.

How can we be so selfish and keep Jesus Christ just for ourselves? We should share Him with everyone that needs Him; He has enough for all of us. Let's all ask him for a little for everyone and that way we would have a different opinion about each other and it would be easier to love one another. Jesus Christ is the answer and the only one, especially for those who are lost and don't have a place to get refuge. We can seek refuge in Jesus, he will give us shelter. He is like a big tree that gives us shade and like a fountain that gives us water to drink. He is the rock that sustains us and He is everything we need. What else can we ask for? He has the answer for everything that bothers us.

It is June already. Time goes by really quickly for me. It hasn't been a good day; one of my patients died today. All his family was here. They looked good people. I was very sad, but at the same time I was happy because I knew he went to Heaven. Before he died, he regretted everything he did and he became closer to God and had Jesus Christ in his heart. He didn't have to suffer anymore; he had better company now and would never have to suffer again. For the rest of us life goes on and we need to keep moving forward until it's our turn.

I'm not very happy today. I had a small issue with one of the nurses. When I got here, she told me she wanted to see me in her office. She told me she didn't want me to talk to my patients about God.

I felt so bad about it that I wasn't able to bring happiness to the people that so much needed spiritual love. I believe in God and I know he performs miracles.

She told me that she didn't believe in God and if I came to her and talk to her about God I would offend her.

I felt like dying.

They were prohibiting me to do the one thing I love in my life. God is good and almighty. How can anyone prohibit you to talk people about God when they are dying? Especially when God is the one thing they have. They are the ones that need Him the most. I'm praying to God to help me take this pain I have inside my chest. Nobody wants to understand, but I know God is with me. Some people don't understand the only thing we need is to have Him on our side. We need to talk about Him to everyone. He is the only one who performs miracles.

Humans were made by God, God was not made by humans, and we need to remember that for the rest of our lives. I don't feel very good today but I give God thanks. I know He is with me and if we were with Him all the time a lot of the things that happen here on Earth wouldn't happen. If you believe in God, you should let Him be since there's people who don't understand Him. Only He understands us and that's all it matters in life. He gives me life and takes it away. I would never get tired of praising His name. He is the one who takes us through the good path.

A lot of people take the wrong path. They engage in drugs, alcohol and many other things. That is how they end up in jail, the hospital or in the cemetery. If we had Jesus Christ in our hearts, none of this would happen.

It is very difficult for to me talk to people, they don't seem to understand or don't want to. Many of them repent when they go to jail but it can be too late, for the rest of the world they are already marked. But if they repent, God gives them a new life even though they are in jail. If you think about it, we are all prisoners of this corrupt, ignorant world. For some people it's easier to hurt others than to help them.

What a horror - this world we live in - corrupt and destructive. I don't know where we are going to end, but saying the truth hurts, what is it we need to say? Lies to make others happy? This it ignorance from our part. To show our love to our neighbor, we should help each other and have love for one another. Everything in life is a sacrifice and nothing is easy or free. I pray to God to give me the strength to continue looking for a place to put all the people that is HIV positive and don't have place to go and need a place to call home.

Is very sad that a lot of them have to die on the streets like dogs because they don't have where to go and nobody loves them. God says that if we do everything He tells us to do, He would give us all the blessings and that's enough for me. I don't think anybody can offer or give us more than Him. When I'm sad I start thinking and I tell myself: "We are nothing." We think life is a game, but it is not. I see my patients every day; I'm with them every day. I don't know how they can take the pain. It is so horrible just to think about it. I asked them how they feel and they tell me its worse than being in hell. This illness can destroy anybody. I feel responsible; we need to help them even if it is just with a little love.

A little love towards them makes such a big difference. I'm saying this out of experience. The majority of these persons never had anybody's love to guide them and teach them what love is about. The majority of the people that are in the hospital or in jail are here because they lack love and no one has taken the time and effort to tell them there is someone out there that loves them.

Nobody is perfect, what I'm trying to say is that if people wouldn't be so liberal and was more charitable we would have less people in places they didn't needed to be. Some people think we are crazy when we are courteous and we are good. We can't forget we are human beings are we make mistakes. I believe we need to treat each other with respect and simplicity.

I'm going back to one of our patients that is not here but in jail. He told me we should have a special place for people HIV positive. They are destined to die and their time is very limited. A place where they can spend the last days of their life, a charming place they can call home. They don't have a place to call home and they are very lonely. Like James - who is HIV positive - and out on the streets with no place to go. That is very painful to me; he is a human being, too.

He has made mistakes. But, how many mistakes have we made? I don't think he wanted to be in this situation, I believe nobody wants to die, especially from this illness. When I talk to him, he gets very happy to know he has someone out there that cares about him. I do what I can for him. I love him very much and he has already suffered so much. He deserves my love. Every day is a different story for him. He is always in his room waiting for death to come. He is always waiting for me to come to work and go talk to him because he has no one else. The rest of the people in the hospital don't have time to talk to him and all the doctors do is give him bad news. He spends his days staring at the walls of his bedroom and when he is done with that he stares at the window. He doesn't know what to do anymore. The only thing he does is smoke. It is the only thing he has left to do. He doesn't have anyone to come see him so his days are truly a burden. He is so alone the only thing he wants to do is die. He doesn't have anyone but he has Jesus, and that's all he needs now. He is no longer alone.

23. Israel, continued.

Israel has been sick for a long time now. This is the third time he came to the hospital. With AIDS you never know when you are going to feel better. He was very depressed, which doesn't help when you have AIDS. I went and spoke with him when I had time and it helped him feel better. He always talked to me about his daughter living in Puerto Rico. He would tell me he would like to see her. It had been a long time since he saw her or heard from her. I told him he would see her again and he replied: 'Of course! I want to get better, get out of jail and go spend time with her. I miss her and I want her to tell me all the things she has done all this time I haven't seen her."

Truth is I felt very sorry for him. He needed someone to give him good advice and comfort. But like many others, he decided to kept himself in that path because that's what felt good at the time. He regretted everything, but now it was too late to change all the things that had happened to him. There was no turning back. It was too late.

What can we do? At least he learned that you don't play with God. Sooner or later we are all going to pay for what we have done. Incredible but true. He told me about where he lived and the things that happened in there. He wasn't very happy with it. Drug after drug; the pain of losing everything. When you are immersed in things you shouldn't be, we should expect the things that happen next. Out of a bad thing you don't get a good one.

He always asked me questions and I responded to him so he didn't felt so alone. He had a very rough life, like many of us, but there are people who know how to get out of the different situations and there are others that have no idea of what they want. In his case, the things that happened to him occurred to him because he was ignorant. What I'm trying to say is that he ignored what would happen to him. And like him, there are millions and millions of people. We don't see it because we are so immerse in our daily tasks that we don't look at the many people who are in need of love and compassion.

Who would have told him that he would've end with AIDS and in jail? Nobody told him about his responsibilities in life. Because of this, he lost his family and his liberty, and everything else he loved in his life.

I think if we spent more time with our children we would help them a little more, none of this would happen. We don't have four eyes and when bad things happen we can't go back. Thank God there are still people out there with good intentions like Magic Johnson, the Basketball player who takes time to teach children what is life about. But he had to get to that situation. If we didn't have people like him we would be all lost. I get very afraid just to think about it. I pray to God that my children learn from all this situations in my book so they can stay in the good path. And if not, is not going to be because I didn't teach them the truth about life.

With all the problems there are in life we never know how our children are going to turn out and this is very sad. I give God thanks because He helps me keep going everyday and mostly because He helps me see the difference between good from bad, which is the most important.

I think we should all unite and do something to avoid this slaughter. Drugs and sex are like a big slaughter. Millions die and many of them are children that don't know anything about life. I don't know where they are going to end. If we don't get savvy with our children they are not going to have any future. The world doesn't give them any alternative. They are helpless against a big monster called AIDS. When they share the syringes with each other they also share the virus - that's how the game begins and that is how it ends. They end in a bed dying like flowers gradually fading away.

I don't believe Israel wanted to end his life this way but for him it's too late. However, for others is not too late if we act quickly.

When Israel figured it out, it was too late. Now, he is buried. That poor girl who loved him so much now she doesn't have a father; she can cry all she wants but that's not going to bring her father back. It is such a cruel experience. Death does not discriminate for age or race; it takes everybody in its path.

HIV takes all the ones who get in its way too, it doesn't forgive anybody. Maybe this will serve as an example for her. She now hates drugs because drugs took away from her the thing she most loved, her father. It is a bad experience; but we can always learn from somebody else's mistakes. It's very hard to learn, is not easy to lose the people we love. Maybe she will continue through the good path and when she is older, gets married and has children, she can teach them about the dangers of drugs and many other things.

I would like to dedicate this part of the book to a dear friend who lost his battle, but I do want everybody to know he will be forever in our hearts. He is now in heaven and before he died he wanted to leave his testimony so others would not make the same mistakes he did while alive. We love you Israel and you will always be within us.

Every night is a new story and new suffering for me because I live with them, suffer with them and cry with them. Their pain is so bad nobody can imagine it. I have children and I would never want to see my children like this; I know how much they suffer and it's something I don't even want to think about it, but they are human and make mistakes like everybody else.

I pray to God I that I'd never have to experience anything like that. I don't think my heart would be able to take the pain, I think I would die but would never abandon them. I would stay with them until the end; they are a very important part of me. They are my blood. If we would only stopped and think about the things that happen around the world and we would have a little more patience, we would take more time to show them the path they need to follow. I think we would save them from a lot of suffering.

We need to remember they are our future and they are a gift from God. If we don't take care of this gift, who that gave it to us has all the right to take it away. I know they are not easy to control but if we don't do it, it's like we would take a gun and put it on their forehead and press the trigger. There is not that much difference between one thing and the other.

This part of the book is dedicated to a boy who fought for his life; he took a piece of my heart with him when he died.

I would like to dedicate this part of the book to a boy who fought against this illness. Not only him, but all of his family. He suffered so much, and I know how much they all suffer because I work with AIDS patients. I can tell you how horrible it is, not only for them, but for their families. Thinking about his mother makes my heart hurt. How can we be so cruel to treat a child this way? Everybody rejected him when he was in school. He didn't have any friends, he only had his parents. That's all he had left. Everybody treat him like a he was a leper, like he was a threat. What a shame! Where is this thing called compassion? What are we - human beings or animals? Not even animals treat their young this way.

I know exactly how he felt, and the bad thing is that I never got to meet him. I would have given all that I have to give him a hug and tell him how much Jesus Christ and I loved him. He was entitled to everything. Just thinking about him fighting the illness puts me at a loss for words. He never had any friends and his parents suffered because others rejected him.

I can imagine how much he suffered because even thought he was only a child; he could feel everything that was happening around him.

He suffered too, they didn't only reject him, and they rejected his family too. I'm sure that was in his mind and I can only imagine the times he asked God to take him with Him. It was like being in hell, nobody can even begin to think how much he suffered, but I do know and I would do anything to give him his life back. He is never going to be able to grow up next to his mom, dad and siblings. It is a shame that nobody gave him the opportunity to express how he really felt. We need to remember that we all have children and only God knows what can happen to them or to us. I wish I would've know him to tell him how valuable he was. It doesn't matter that he didn't knew me; you don't need to know somebody to tell them you love them.

I hope he is in heaven; I would like to hug him, kiss him and tell him how much I love him when I get there. I would've loved to meet him before, when he really needed me. I can only ask God to bless that family. What he and his family suffered, I can't change, but maybe he can serve us as an example. There are many others like him, let's not do the same thing we did to him.

The only thing they ask from us is for us to have compassion and love for them not only for them, but for their families also. They all suffer. I can see it every day because I work with them and I know what it is to be next to them and see them die and not being able to do anything other than let them know their not alone.

They return the favor by giving me a kiss and a hug. I offer them my shoulder, where they rest their heads and cry until they don't have any more tears. My heart is filled with pain and my arms are not big enough for all of them. They are so many that I don't know what I'm going to do with all this suffering and this pain. All this kills me inside, but what can I do?

We need more people to help with AIDS patients. We should always think about that child who fought the battle and lost. I can imagine he felt alone, his life ahead of him and already fighting death when he hadn't started living yet. What an experience he had. And on top of that, he couldn't even go to school like the other children, they all made fun of him and none of the mothers wanted to even see him. I can imagine his suffering, I'm sure he wanted to play with the other children and have a normal life with his family.

I can only ask God to put love in our hearts and that He can make us more compassionate and make us understand that we all make mistakes in our lives. We should be even more compassionate when it is a human life.

All I ask if that whoever reads this book to think about it and understand that there are more people in the same situation this child was in and there is still time to help others. I am going to spend the rest of my life helping others. They need all the love and compassion they can get. If you have a heart, you should do what you can, too. They deserve it after all the suffering. We should not turn our backs on them like we did with this child. I always think of him and all the things he had to go through. We need to consider ourselves very fortunate that we don't have to go through what he had to live.

I have three children and I hope I've never have to go through a situation like that. It is horrible to see how their bodies die a little bit every day and you can't do anything. It is really painful, and I can only pray for them. Nobody knows what they go through but we can make their lives less painful and happier. They really need it. Sometimes I start wondering what would you do if you had a child with AIDS and the other children didn't wanted to play with him and they would neglect him, throw stones and your window and damn you. I think that would really hurt us. But, when that child is not ours, we don't care.

That is not right, they are innocent and they didn't ask to have HIV. Those are things that happen in life and we need to learn how to deal with them and learn to respect the people that have AIDS because the you never know when it can be you in that situation. I know to never say never, I don't know what destiny has for me and we should always be alert in case one day, God helps us. We need to deal with this.

Everything is possible; we are not excluded of having a bad experience. If something like that would happen to us we need to be prepared. Like I said before – you never know what destiny will bring to you.

Where I work the majority of the patients have AIDS. Each night is worse than the other. If you could only see how much they suffer, cry and scream asking for mercy and asking to die constantly. If you only knew how many of them ask me to take their life away. This is a suffering that I have constantly in my heart.

Some of them go blind and can't eat by themselves or can't see what they have on their plate. They depend on someone to help them with their food and drinks. They need someone to make their beds or read them the Bible. We are their eyes; they can't do anything for themselves, and that makes them feel alone. They need someone to talk to, since they can only hear and talk. Some of them have different symptoms like memory loss, hair loss and some look like they are in a vegetative state. It is a never-ending story.

Maybe one day they will find the cure for this illness, it is really hard to know that you are dying but you can do anything; just wait for that day to come. It is very sad; they don't have anything else on what to spend their time other than counting the minutes they have left. It is so sad to see them this way, like they are lost; with hope for nothing with an empty look in their eyes.

They look everywhere but not really looking for anything, like they are looking for something they lost but don't know where to find it. It is one thing to describe it to you and another to be there and experience it with them. This is a terrible illness; it starts from one point and doesn't end until you die. It is a real trauma that you don't really know what to do to help them with their suffering, but everything is possible with love. There is a little relief for their bodies if we give them some love. Here, where I work, it is really sad; even thought I would like to do more I can't.

My health is not very good and they are always making us work so much, we are always short on people. I have 26 patients and I have to take care of all of them. The only one who can really help them is God. God is the only one that can help me take away this pain I have inside me, I do suffer a lot with them.

To deal with people who have AIDS can be very difficult. You need to know how to treat them and how to understand them. When they feel depressed, we need to be very careful because they can be dangerous. They know they are dying and don't care about anything. They don't care if they hurt one or 40. I've seen some patients get violent and slap the nurses. Usually this happens when the patient is confused or somebody has made him mad. This doesn't happen much.

What we need to have is a lot of understanding and patience; they are so sick they don't even want to look at themselves. This could be very painful; we don't even know how to react. We need to help them keep going; they are like children that don't know how to get out of the situation. This is very serious, if we weren't so arrogant and vain we would see things a different way.

24. James, continued.

James continues in the hospital and it looks like every day that goes by he gets worse. He always calls me and asks me for a cigarette. He is losing a lot of weight and is starting to look like a strand of spaghetti. He doesn't want to eat. I have learned so much from him, like he always says; sometimes we take things for granted.

When I talk to him, he tells me about his life and how his friends would take his food and money when he was out living in the streets. Those were not friends really, but even if they were, none of them come to the hospital to see him.

He gets really happy when he sees me get to work because he knows I'm going to go see him and give him a cigarette. The most important thing is that I talk with him and that makes his life much better. He knows that when he needs me I will go see him. He needs to talk to somebody. There are many others like him; he doesn't have any family but the most important thing is that he has Jesus in his heart and he has me and my family and that makes him really happy. I think about him when I'm by myself.

He is slowly dying and he knows it. He tells me he doesn't care anymore because he doesn't have anybody in this world. The only thing he has received in here is insults, nobody to comfort him. For him, life has been sad and long and I know it's true. You only need to look at his face to know this is true. He would've loved to have a mom and a dad and grow up in a home like the other children and play with his siblings. To have many other things we have and take for granted and even if they are small things, he would've loved to have them anyway.

Sometimes the little things are what matter, but who pays attention to the little things? Usually people go for the big stuff. I believe we need to pay attention to small things, that way when we get bigger things we can deal with it. I talk to him about many other things.

He gets really happy to know I have a mom and a dad who love me very much and they have always given me love and continue to do it. They have taught me to show and expect respect, and to help others when they need it. I am really proud of them; they've always given me good advice. I'm happy that God gave me a family like the one I have. It's sad that I have so much and he doesn't have anything. There is nothing we can do, just survive the best we can. I pray to God to give me the opportunity to make him understand that there are millions like him.

Even here in New York, all you have to do is look outside on the streets and what do you see? Destruction, immorality, crime, drugs, etc. The majority of the people who haven't had an education like we have, only God knows why that is, they are all abandoned to drugs and they don't care about killing, rapping, hitting or insulting anybody who gets in their way. They don't know what they are doing, but nobody cares to find out why they get that way. I think we would never know, specially knowing we are not interested in anybody. Maybe one day we will understand why; if we take the time to get to know them better.

For the majority of them, the only thing they need is a friend and good advice. I feel badly for them when I see them out in the streets. Most have children, and those poor children are born with HIV and addicted to drugs.

God, what a horrible crime, nobody knows what that is about and we will probably never will since we only care about ourselves. Pretty much all of the ones that are out in the streets have AIDS and don't know it, and the ones that know it go out with anyone and they don't care. They know they are going to die so they want to take others with them. They don't care who they infect, they just want to gain money with somebody else's blood. It is a terrible sin that humanity likes to gain money to buy things this way.

This is a crime that has no forgiveness from God. Money is the cause of all bad things, money eats people's lives. . It doesn't matter how much money they have, they can't buy the cure for AIDS.

In here, every person is a different story and without us knowing they can ask for help but we can't see it. We don't pay attention to anything but ourselves, but if we would slow down and listen to their story we would be happier to have what we have. It is like the world has gone crazy, all these sickness, we think that things are going to get better but that's not the case and we don't want to recognize it. Children these days have more liberty, are not respectful and don't want to listen to their parents. Don't even mention going to church - they don't want anything to do with that - it's as if they are allergic.

All they want to do is listen to their music and live the good life while we worry about them. The advice we give them doesn't work, if they would do what we tell them, I'm sure they won't be so many with AIDS.

I don't know what to do, there are parents who abuse their children; this has no forgiveness either. There is no respect anymore; the government spends money on weapons while others don't have anything to eat or where to live. Everytime I think about it, it makes less sense to me. We are not here forever so we need to be more adjusted to reality and less materialistic. One of these days, we would find the answer to all of this that is happening; I just hope is not too late for a lot of people. For some it is already too late because they are dead, but there is nothing we can do about that; what we can is help the ones that are alive.

25. Johnson's story

Tonight has been a horrible night. We had two patients die. AIDS has stolen two more lives. The more I think about it, the less I know how to feel. Every day is worse here at the hospital. We have, many patients in very advanced stages of AIDS, and it feels like they all die at the same time. I started my night like every other night. I took care of all my patients and then went to see my friend Johnson. He is very sick. When I got into his room I said hello and stayed talking with him for a long time.

I went to check his temperature and when I did, he started having convulsions. I didn't know what was going on so I started screaming and calling the nurses. When the nurse arrived she told me not worry about it, that it was nothing. But my eyes couldn't stop staring at him. I told the nurse that he was dying because he wasn't breathing. She took his pulse and became really nervous. It was then that I realized he was dead. He died quickly, before we could realize it. I was in total shock; five minutes before I was talking with him.

We prepared to send him to the morgue for an autopsy where they would cut him in into pieces to send to the cemetery. Just thinking about it gives me goose bumps, but I need to be strong and keep going; there are many other patients that need me. This one doesn't need me anymore.

26. John's story

Half an hour after another one died. His name was John; he was here for six months and it really surprised me that he lasted this long. He was always screaming in pain. He was a very rude patient that would insult me and everyone else in the hospital. He did it to me many times but I resented him. He was dying. I always treated him with respect and didn't care about his insults.

All those months in agony, only God knows how much he suffered, he never accepted that he had AIDS. He was upset with everybody; like it was our fault he had AIDS.

It is very hard for some people to deal with the fact they have AIDS. Only a few can deal with it. There is nothing we can do for them, only to help them and to pray for them. They need a spiritual guide; only when they are dying they want to be close to God.

John was very skinny because he refused to eat and many other things. He looked like a skeleton. This is normal in here; they go through so many treatments and experiments that when they die they are only skin and bones. John had a very particular way of being, he always insulted me each time he saw me but I didn't care because I knew he was dying, but deep inside it did bother me because I had always been very nice to him. He always treated me like a dog. I forgive him; he just wanted me to suffer.

That made him happy; he always started laughing after he insulted anybody.

Here at the hospital I have two nurses that are driving me crazy, they don't give me a break. There is a lot of work to do in the hospital and I don't stop all night. Walking all night from one room to the other. Working like a slave and they are just sitting in there doing nothing. I have to deal with 26 patients and on top of that they complain. It's like a mad house in here. The hospital doesn't really want to spend more money on bringing more nurses but we really need help. At least the patients really like me because I treat them well, if I treated them badly I'm sure they wouldn't wanted to see me.

We had a patient here that the doctor gave 48 hours to live. That night, he called me to his room and said this to me:

"Josefina, thank you for making me so happy and for treating me like a human being, for being here when I most needed it. I thank you with all my heart. Thanks for making me smile and for giving me a shoulder to cry on. Thank you for all the moments where you made me feel like a person without asking anything in return. God bless you."

I thought I was dreaming, all of that was a surprise for me and I didn't know what to do so I gave him a kiss and a hug and said goodbye. He didn't want to die without saying those things to me and that made me feel so bad. I knew he appreciated me and I appreciate him. I learned a lot from him; he knew he was dying and was so confident. I went to see him a couple of times that night, we knew he wasn't going to make it pass that night. I saw how his life was slowly going off. I don't know what he was thinking but he looked confused, like he was at a train station waiting for the train to come, but doesn't want the train to come because he doesn't want to go away. His became more and more confused. He didn't understand what was happening, he only knew his life was ending and he needed to put his ideas in order.

Only God knows what he had inside his mind. It was like nothing was important for him anymore, he just sat on his bed counting the days, the minutes and the seconds he had left until he die. Death came and he was ready for it. He just took a breath of air and then he was gone. It was over for him. His family was there with him, they looked all lost; they knew they were going to lose a much loved family member and they knew they were never going to see him again.

It is like fighting a battle that has no ending; they fight with all their strength for something is already a lost cause. You can see the pain in the relatives faces; you can tell of all the pain and all the sleepless nights. When they die, you see a different face, like when you are giving birth and after all that suffering and pain the baby is born dead.

They asked themselves - Have we lost the battle? There is nothing else to do but pick up the pieces because the families are now shattered. This illness causes you to wish you were never born; it is incredible. We need to realize that when it's all over there is nothing for us to do. Unfortunately, there are many others sick still alive and going through the same path. The only thing we can do is pray for them. They have no cure for their illness and it's really hard to comprehend how they feel because we are not inside their heads. If we paid more attention to them, we would be able to understand them. They are human beings and deserve understanding and love. With everything they go through it's no wonder they get depressed. They go through a lot of pain and many other things. Sometimes a small detail can make all the difference, they appreciate the small details much more than big things. I think about the things that make them happy all the time. They have so little time left that they can't really enjoy the details. Some of them realize how much better their lives could've been if they didn't have AIDS, but it is too late now. They remember their mistakes and even though it is too late to go back, they can recognize their mistakes. Better late than never.

Sometimes I try to put myself in their place but it is not the same, I'm not the one dying so it's really difficult for me. I still understand them and respect them. They have no other choice than to wait for death to come get them. The majority of them are prisoners so their lives are full of stories, each of them incredible. I think about it and I give God thanks I was raised in a good environment with good parents that always cared for me and gave me everything I needed.

My mom always said to me that I needed to respect everything that wasn't mine and if we needed something we needed to ask her and not just take it. We grew up in a nice environment. I think about it and thank God for the parents I have. It is a blessing for me; I'll never be going to be able to repay to them everything they did for me. My mother gave us a good education and the only thing I can say is that I'm eternally grateful for everything they did for me, my brothers and my sisters. I hope they do the same for their children. A lot depends on how we treat them so they can learn to be nice. I would like for my children to be decent, educated people and never to hurt anyone. I have educated them differently so they can respect others; if they start having bad acquaintances that's how they'll end too.

Many of them don't know what it is to love and be loved; they have been raised by abusive people and most of them live on the streets. Others have been raised by a single mom that has to work to two jobs in order to support them. That is not easy, and I know this by experience, when the mother is working the children will do bad things. They start hanging around the wrong people that only want to know what they can get from them. They give those drugs and many other things.

Once they become drug users, they have no other way but to start stealing to keep the vice that will be the beginning of their end. As time goes by, they need more and more and they start stealing bigger and bigger things to keep their habit. At some point, they go out to steal and kill. Drugs have complete control over their lives and if they have to kill someone to get them they don't care; drugs have them completely dominated.

They have told me stories that had given me goose bumps of how horrible they are. The majority of prisoners we have here have started this way and they end here at the hospital; with HIV without even believing for one second they were going to end this way. Some of them end here at the hospital, some at the cemetery. I don't believe we give birth to our children to give them away to this monster that is AIDS.

It is not easy to put them inside the plastic bags when they die. It is not like putting meat in the freezer. But, it is my job and I have to do it.

Who knows if one day I'll be the one inside the plastic bag? It's a hard job, but I always make sure I help them when they are alive.

My job is my first priority, before everything else just comes along, even my health. They need me and I'm here to help and that makes me happy. It is an honor for me to be able to care for them. They are very sick and need someone to care for them. A lot of the people here do it for the money, not for the patients. They don't care if they are dying or if their head hurts. They don't want to waste their time with them and some use a foul language with them. At the end, we all pay the consequences of what we do to others.

27. James, continued.

James, after being here for a long time and suffering a great deal, has died. His battle is over, he would not suffer anymore, and he is now with God. He is now healthy and in heaven but I still miss him so much. He doesn't need me anymore, but there are other patients that do. Every time I think of him I miss him and it's so hard when they die, it's like a fairy tale that never has a happy ending.

The only thing I ask God is to end with AIDS. There are many others who are going to end the same way the ones here. This is like coming back from Vietnam. I have their faces inside my head and I can't take them away doesn't matter how much I try. I can't really do much by myself, but like my mother always says: "Together we can all achieve more" I think that if we get together we can really do something for them but we need to start right away, too many have die already and keep dying every day that goes by.

This is something that concerns all of us. If things keep going this way, we can all end like them or worse. Who knows if it can happen to our children? Nobody is exempt to this illness. Sometimes I ask myself how with all this science and they still haven't found a cure.

I think they are trying, but we are almost to the point of giving up. Every day that goes by is harder for me to get used to all these situations. My patients ask me if we have found a cure for AIDS and I don't know what to tell them. It is heartbreaking to see them like this. God said to us: 'Love your brother like you love yourself," but how can we do this if we don't know how to care for ourselves?

It sounds ridiculous but it is true. Every day I see how many hypocrites we have around us. They act very friendly when in front of you but when you turn your back they destroy you. I see it a lot in the hospital, they all think are superior to you and if you don't follow their games you are not good enough.

I feel much better when I'm with my patients; I know they appreciate what I do for them with all their heart. They are all very important to me and I do what I do with love, I know they need me and need my understanding and love. Most of them are rejected by their families and friends because they are afraid they may get infected. What does he have to look forward in life? Just wait until it is time to die?

It is really painful to see them like this, with nothing and no one to help you or count on, really sad. Not even dogs deserve to be treated like that and that's why I love them so much. God tells us to help the ones that need it, and the people that have HIV need it the most. We should all get motivated and help them; you never know when it is going to be you needing the help. We need each other; if we only thought of all the things we have but we don't give any importance but they are never going to get we would understand how fortunate we really are.

28. Mark's story

Today I was thinking of a patient that died two weeks ago. His name was Mark. I use to talk to him a lot, he would tell me about his life and all the things he used to do. He was very afraid of dying. I used to talk to him about the things he did. Now he could remember everything because he knew he didn't had a lot of time left. After a couple days, his memory wasn't that good anymore. He couldn't even remember the things we had talked about days before. That seem to bother him a lot and sometimes he just stayed quiet. I tried not to pay too much attention to it, I knew what was going on and didn't want to alarm him. I just kept talking to him that seemed to make him happy. He would tell me of all the things he was going to do when he got out of the hospital. He had a lot of plans but didn't realize that he was just daydreaming and these were the last hours alive. I wasn't going to tell him. I wanted him to feel as comfortable as he could; that is my job - make his days as comfortable as possible.

The only thing he had left now was wait to die. Sometimes he would tell me things that made me cry because I knew he was crying. Every time I entered his room he called me by my name. There were days his mind was clear and some other days it wasn't, but he always remembered my name. That's a very rare thing. Days kept going by, and he kept getting worst. He needed to have surgery but because he was so sick the doctors were too afraid to do it. They didn't want to take any risks;

they knew he was dying so there was no point in putting him through surgery. He lasted much longer than what doctors expected. He really was fighting to survive. He didn't wanted to die even thought he knew he was dying.

His last days were really sad, he looked terrible and that was very painful for me, knowing I couldn't do anything for him. Only God knows what it is to suffer that way, I don't think any of us would ever understand and I wish I'd never have to experience anything like this.

I can only think about his poor mother. Watching his son die and suffer like this. That must be a very painful thing, seeing your son suffer and not even knowing how to handle it. Seeing AIDS take away the person you had inside you and you raised for 20 years. It's must be very sad.

I'm a mother, too, and I know how much I would suffer if I had to go through something like this with any of my children.

He died today; his mother just lost her child, the child that she took care of night after night, fed, bathed, loved, covered when he was cold, and took care of when he was sick. All those years gone in a second, and now she cries for the son the world has taken away from her. There is nothing like a mother's love for her children. Who is going to bring her son back? Who is going to console her and tell her that everything is going to be all right? Who is going to pick up the pieces of that broken heart? Only God can make that miracle happen. We can help, too, by not letting our children fall down this path. The world will offer them everything but is only a trick to make them fall for it and then don't let them go until there is nothing left out of them.

Little by little the world will immerse them into drugs, sex, and alcohol. All those things come along with drugs. I think is time for us to unite and protest against drugs. It is taking our children away and we are not even realizing it. They don't only rob our children, they also rob us of all those years of happiness we could've had. We need to do something before it's too late. Pretty soon, we are not going to be able to do anything. Everyday that goes by is worse with more drugs, crime and the number one enemy - AIDS.

God help us.

Wake up and realize they are robbing us our children, something that belongs to us. They are like gold to us and no one has any right to come get them from us. Only God knows how we are going to end. It is proven that we can't trust humanity. Some people would steal your brain if they could just to get one dollar. It is sad how little value life has when it should be the most precious thing. I wish I could change things, but I can't do miracles. If only some of us would get together I'm sure we could change many of the things that are happening. I know we can't get back the ones that already died, but we can help the ones that need us. Long before they die, they do suffer a lot when they are in prison and that's really sad because the vast majority is good children.

God, what is happening in this world? Most of us are either crazy or blind.

There are a lot of people out in the streets with AIDS. Some of them know it, others don't. The ones that don't have an excuse, but the ones that have it and just spread it don't deserve to be forgiven by God.

They are sentencing all those people to die. They probably think that if they are dying, why not take others with them? We need to be very careful, some people don't look like they have AIDS, but they do. You never know who is a carrier of the virus so we need to understand that if we have too many sex partners we can wake up with surprises.

It is not an easy thing to relate to when you tell someone they have AIDS. It's like telling them: "you are dying". This is the reality of life; you can trust no one today. This is why is so important to be cautious, anybody can make a mistake.

When they show on TV a person with AIDS, it doesn't look bad at all. What they don't show is when they are covered in sores and they look like skeletons or when they start throwing up blood.

I don't want to keep going; it makes me nauseous just to think about it. They show a nice version on TV, but they reality is much worse than you can imagine. It's like a horror movie and everyday that goes by we have more and more people with AIDS. It's like a plague than when it starts you don't know when it's going to end. My worst two years as a nurse have been the ones working with them, all that pain they go through, no one can really understand it.

I do know it too because I've been with them two years already and sometimes I have wished to die with them. An illness that consumes them day after day and not being able to do anything for them is even worse because they are always on my mind.

It's like they are in hell and they are torturing them every day. This is something that concerns us all and we need to raise our voice and do something, somebody is going to hear us. They have already suffered enough and the worst thing is that there is no exit. The only thing left to do is pray and ask God to help us get out of this epidemic. It looks easy from the outside but is really not.

We need to reconsider and start seeing things a different way, they are human beings after all. The way things are going right now, I don't think we are going to have space for them; everybody is terrorized with this illness. I can't blame them, but that doesn't mean we need to put them out of our way because we are afraid of getting it.

Who is going to take care of them? Before we make a decision we need to think about it. If we abandon them, who is going to take care of them? They don't have anybody to help them. I pray every day that more people would be willing to help them. It is a shame they don't have anybody and are so lonely. Most of them haven't had someone that can make them happy in all their lives. They have suffered all their lives and now they don't have anybody that can take care of them. I'm the kind of person that, because of this I may have very few friends and a lot of enemies, but I feel it necessary to help the ones that need it.

If we only follow Jesus Christ example, he taught us so many things. We need to read about his life and see how he used all his life to help others. If we decided to do the same things we are different, but we don't. We need to help the ones that need it because AIDS doesn't respect race, color or age.

It doesn't matter what religion, it's like a hungry piranha that eats everything that gets in its way. AIDS is an illness that always wins. Be very careful with it. Open your eyes about what AIDS is doing to us; it's an enemy that attacks from behind without giving us an opportunity to defend ourselves.

A person with AIDS needs love and understanding. They are rejected by everybody and become depressed. There are many things we can't understand because is not us in the situation. I always ask for their opinion when I talk to the AIDS patients.

It's very important we understand you don't get AIDS from the toilet seat or by getting in a pool or by using the same glass. We need to keep helping them as much as we can because only God knows how much they suffer.

29. Henry's story

Just today another one died another one to add to the AIDS count. His name was Henry. This was his third time here, but this time he stayed forever. I remember talking to him only a few times, he was very private and well educated. He was also a prisoner. I always asked him if he needed anything, but it was like he didn't want to bother anyone. His family never came to visit him and that made me really sad because he looked so lonely. His loneliness was even worse because he had no one to talk to. Who was he going to tell how lonely and depressed he was? Maybe if he would've had someone next to him things would've been a little better, knowing his family was on his side. We will never know why they never came to visit. He died alone, with no one on his side. This makes me sad because I don't think anybody would like to die alone like that. At least he won't suffer anymore now. He didn't talked much so I don't know what kind of person he was but he looked like a nice one but with a lot of problems.

Every day that goes by I understand them a little better. They all have pretty much the same history. They don't know how they started on drugs or how, the only thing they know is that they are there and don't know how to get out. They do know how they are going to end. The majority of them has AIDS and knows that sooner or later they are going to end like all the other ones. I ask God to help me because I have three children and you never know how they are going to end. If we can only help them in any way we could we would be doing something very generous and they do need it. Another one that lost the battle with AIDS and I ask myself how many others are going die? I think many more. Every day we have more AIDS related deaths. Many of them don't have anybody and don't know what to do and become desperate.

Often people make fun of me and ask me why I like to work with them and why I treat them well. I can't change it; it hurts me so much to see them suffer like this. Is not my fault I was born this way? Maybe with God's help I may be able to open a place where I can take care of them. This is the purpose of the book. I will continue to do everything I can to help them because to me is worth something. Even if it is to keep them company and to help them move forward until the day they die. They die a little bit every day. Some of them handle it well, others not so much. We are all going to die, we are not immortal.

I just don't want to die of AIDS because it's horrible all they have to go through, like it never ends. They can only rest when they die. Then, everything is over. You will never know how much one suffers with these people. When they get depressed and lonely they think about suicide but I can't really do much because I don't know what it is to be in their situation. The only thing I can do for them is help them spiritually and morally. I can try to understand them and make the time they have left comfortable. If people would only know half of the stuff they need to know about this illness, things would be different because they would at least try to help them. But, because no one has taken the time to teach us or figure out how much they can really hurt us, we don't want anything to do with them.

Just by hearing HIV it's like hearing "leper". You can't get AIDS by touching the patient. If we would just take a little bit of time to learn about this illness, we would know that you can't get AIDS that easily. But, it is easier to be ignorant and not find out the why and how. This is really a shame and it doesn't have any excuse to be like that. I have taken the time to learn about this illness and that's why I work with them. It really hurts me to see them being rejected like dogs. But until we learn all of this we would never know how they feel and how they think.

30. Ricky's story

We have a really young guy in C4 in here. He is 26 years old and he is dying. There is no remedy for Ricky. I know God doesn't mind that they are dying, he loves them anyway and his love is enough. It's very painful to have to pay for the sins we have committed but what really hurts is to have everybody against us. What is done is done.

We should let it go and do what we can now because you never know when AIDS is going to be at your door. What are we going to tell it, to come tomorrow because today we are not ready? I'm really trying to get across that we are all confused; this illness is really taking people lives. Why is it so hard to talk about it with our children and tell them of all the consequences it brings? We should take the time and explain to them about all the consequences of AIDS. We should explain to them about the results that this illness can bring for all the relatives. It looks like in today's world there is no space for our children, and we need to make sure we do everything possible to guide them right. They can be naive and be influenced by the wrong people.

I have been talking with some people that are in prison and have AIDS, they have told me it is like being in hell. The flames and the pain never ends, it burns you constantly. I have seen the results of AIDS, and they really are disastrous. The worst thing is that there is no cure for it. They have to live their lives like that until they die, all the time in pain.

I don't know how they move forward, it's really hard to accept that you are dying and not being able to react to it.

Many of them try to be brave and that helps them, some others can deal with it and the first thing they think of is suicide. Some of them live longer than others, some of them start reading the Bible and that helps them. They think of God and the wonders he created and that makes them feel better. Others just get in bed and just wait for death to come get them. They don't want to talk or hear about God. They blame Him for their illness.

The reality is God didn't tell them to go do bad things; they don't want to recognize it thought. They just stay in bed and decide not to fight it because they want to die as soon as possible to stop suffering. It is not easy to have AIDS, what happens is that some of them still wanted to live even though they are dying. I pray to God to find the way to help them in whatever way possible, because they are dying but there is always an opportunity for us to help them. Here at the hospital, the only thing they do with them is use them for experiments. I have seen things in this hospital that I don't even want to mention. Some people lose the ability to walk due to all the injections they have had in their spine. Others throw up their stomachs due to all the pills they give them. This causes them to become anemic and many other things.

It's really hard sometimes, they ask me questions and I don't know what to tell them. What am I going to tell them, that they are dying? They know that already. What they need is somebody to help them keep going. They are already depressed and the doctors won't tell them anything. Test after test and they can't really do anything about it. They need all the support they can get from us.

I'd had the opportunity to speak with many of the relatives and I have had some very interesting conversations. They know how to react and they are aware of all the consequences of the illness. They know they are not going to get infected so it is easier for them to deal with the patient. They understand them and help them the best way they can. They love them, understand them and do the most they can for them.

I'm happy because I had the opportunity of talking to them about God; they need God in moments like this. It is the only thing they have left now.

Some of them didn't even know God existed and now they have dedicated their lives to serve Him. I thank God for giving me this job and the opportunity to love this people who need so much love and understanding.

We have a patient who was been here three or four months and all this time I've been with keeping him company and talking to him about the many mistakes he made.

As we all know the world can offer us so many things but we need to stay strong and with our heads clear. He was telling me how he got to that extreme with drugs and how much he regrets it now, that if God helps him get out of this one he would never touch drugs again. He now understands that what he did was so stupid and now he is paying the consequences of his mistakes. Now it's too late to go back, so he wants to do what's right. God is fair and he would make us pay for what we did before. He would like to start a new life, be a good person and enjoy what he has left of his life. Look only forward because the past is gone and he can't go back to that. All these months he's being with us he has gotten a little bit better.

Now he wants to recover all the time that he lost being on drugs. He couldn't even think when he was using drugs. Now, it looks like he is finally clean and wants to do all he can to keep going. He has told me all the things that happened to him when he injected himself with all the drugs. Now, the only way for him to stay clean is to be good and wait for his turn to die. I was talking with him today and he doesn't look good. They are giving him a very strong medicine and he is not feeling well.

The good thing is that he is in peace with God. He is not afraid of dying, he knows he is going to heaven and you can tell he has that peace that he never had.

Sometimes we need to go to the extreme of seeing ourselves dying to understand we are nothing. Now the only thing he can do its wait, but God is always with him and He would go with him no matter what happens. He has suffered enough already and his mistakes have cost him a very high price to pay. He is not alone, I go see him every night and talk to him. He asks me to read the Bible to him or sometimes he would read it himself and so on. We take turns and let time go by. That's what's really important for me, to know he is having a good time in the short time he has to live. The only problem is that he has too much time to think.

He's like a little boy. Sometimes I look at him and it breaks my heart to know he doesn't have anybody by his side and he is going to die alone. Sometimes he tells me all the things he did while he was out in the streets and how he realizes that he shouldn't had been doing those things. I told him that he didn't needed to worry about it, we all make mistakes and for some of us it doesn't even get to our conscience. He is not the only one that had made mistakes.

This is a very special night for both of us; he has accepted Jesus Christ in his heart. He is no longer afraid of dying. He now is in peace with God and that's the only thing that matters for him and for me. He would like for me and my family to become his friends when he gets out of the hospital. I have told him that that it is not a problem. I told him we would take him on trips to wherever he wanted.

He doesn't have any friends, all the people he knows is involved with drugs. He needs good friends that keep his mind occupied so he doesn't have to think about his illness, to help him keep moving forward and to understand him.

Every time we talk, we have very interesting conversations. For some reason, we always end up talking about the same thing, HIV. Sometimes when I'm by myself I think of the things we talk and I start wondering how they must feel knowing they are dying and there's nothing they can do. It must be very sad and depressing but we would never know because we are not in their place. Sometimes I think of the things they are missing, like to go out and enjoy all the different things God has made. They miss the flowers, birds, the sea and the land. Things that we don't really give any importance to, but they are never going to be able to enjoy because their lives are so fragile.

I get sick to my stomach thinking of all those people who made money selling drugs thinking money is going to buy them happiness. Just to think about it makes me nauseous; they haven't seen the results that their drugs have caused. How wrong they are - money just brings them destruction and at the end they all end up the same way. If they knew what HIV is, they would think it twice about what they do and how much they suffer.

I hope if they read this book they can end with this monster and get away from it. There are so many dying today, and not only adults, little children too; who are paying the consequences of what adults have done. Children are sentence to death even before they start living. I don't know why they have to pay for the mistakes we had made. They didn't ask to come to this world. It should be different for them, they should have the love from their parents and all those things babies have but they never will because they are born with a mark.

A lot of people think AIDS causes death, but before death there's the torture and the pain the body suffers when they can't take it anymore and then they die.

Their bodies shake like they have just being shocked with an electric charge and their stomachs erupt like volcanoes, always throwing up. Their bodies all covered in sores and bleeding. They are so skinny they look like marine algae when they move, so fragile like they are going to break just by looking at them.

When AIDS is finally done with them it looks like Hitler just tortured them. Eyes closed shut, dry from all the tears and in so much pain all they do is scream and ask God to take them away soon. Their hands are shaking all the time; they can't hold anything. Their throats get dry, they get narrow to the point they can not eat or drink. They feel like they have fire in their stomachs. They feel alone and desperate waiting for someone to hug them and tell them they love them and I'm here for you. Their veins get dry like sea plants when the tide goes down, they lose their nails like when a tree looses it leaves. Leaves that go away and never come back. Their hair is like when corn starts to get in season and looses all the fuzz at the top. Their teeth are like a cheap dress that you buy and start getting discolored.

It's like they go through the four seasons until all they have left is their leaves on the floor to them inside a plastic bag. Now to the trash and both the leaves and their bodies would be dust again. From dust we are all made.

How much pain I feel when I see all this going on. It's like having a thorn in your heart all the time. God knows how much I have suffered, you can't even begin to imagine all the ones that have died in my arms. It is a pain so big is almost heavy to carry on. Most of them end on the cemetery; some are less fortunate and end up at a medical tests table. All divided in little pieces, their bodies are to never able to find the rest they deserve. It's like they are in a meat market where they sell meat pieces. Their bodies are all around the table for them to look for God knows what. Not even dead can they rest.

I ask myself, what is it that they look inside their bodies? I never know of the results of their investigations.

God is the only one that has the answer to all the questions we are looking for, they are never going to find the answer they are looking for, and God is the only one that has all the answers.

Doctors don't make miracles, they are human beings and make mistakes like we all do and there are things that continue to be a mystery for them. Many times the experiments can cost someone's life. We are not supposed to know this, and they cover each other very well.

Like they always say, this is the law of life, whoever is born must eventually die. It is one thing to die when it's your turn, and another to have someone take your life like that because of a mistake they made. They are not perfect and make a lot of mistakes and the patients pay this with their lives.

Only God knows when this monster – HIV - that is taking away so many lives is going to end. I hear a lot of things at the hospital and

I think, if they are already dying, why torture them even more with all that medicine and tubes all over their bodies? Instead of all this experiments they should give them pain medication and let them die with dignity. This is the only thing they want.

They inject so many things on them their arms look like colanders with no more space to add another injection. Sometimes I don't even comprehend all of this, like a bad dream that has no end and we are trapped in it. I don't think anybody asks to have HIV, and we all make mistakes but this is a very high price to pay for it. They suffer a lot and at the end they pay with their lives.

Instead of criticizing them we should help them in every way we can, like God has asked us to do. We all have sinned and broken one of the Ten Commandments. The loneliness they feel makes them die before its time and that time they have left is so precious it's a shame to throw it all away like that.

God said: "Not only from bread lives the man, but with what I have gave him to eat and drink spiritually" In order for them to continue forward they need to hear God's word. Many of them don't even remember Him until they are dying. They ask "Why me God?" But God didn't choose this lifestyle for us, we did and now we pay the consequences.

Here I have a poem Israel wrote to me before he died and I would like to share it with all of you:

The Bible contains the mind of God, the state of the man, the way of salvation, the doom of sinners and the happiness of the believers. Its doctrines are holy, its precepts are binding, and it's immutable. Read it to be wise, believe it to be safe, and practice to be holy. It contains light to direct you, food to support you and comfort to cheer you. It is the travelers map, the pilgrim's staff, the pilots compass, the soldier's sword and the Christian's charter. Here paradise is restored, heaven opened and the gates of hell disclosed. Amen. Christ is its big subject, for our good design, and the glory of God its end. It should fill the memory, rule the heart and guide the feet. Read it slowly, frequently and prayerfully. It is mine of wealth. A paradise of glory and a river of pleasure, it is given you in life, will be opened on judgment day, and be remembered forever. It involves the highest responsibility, will reward the greatest labor and will condemn all who trifle with is sacred contents, Amen.

Righteousness exalts a nation but sin is a reproach to any people - Proverbs 14:34

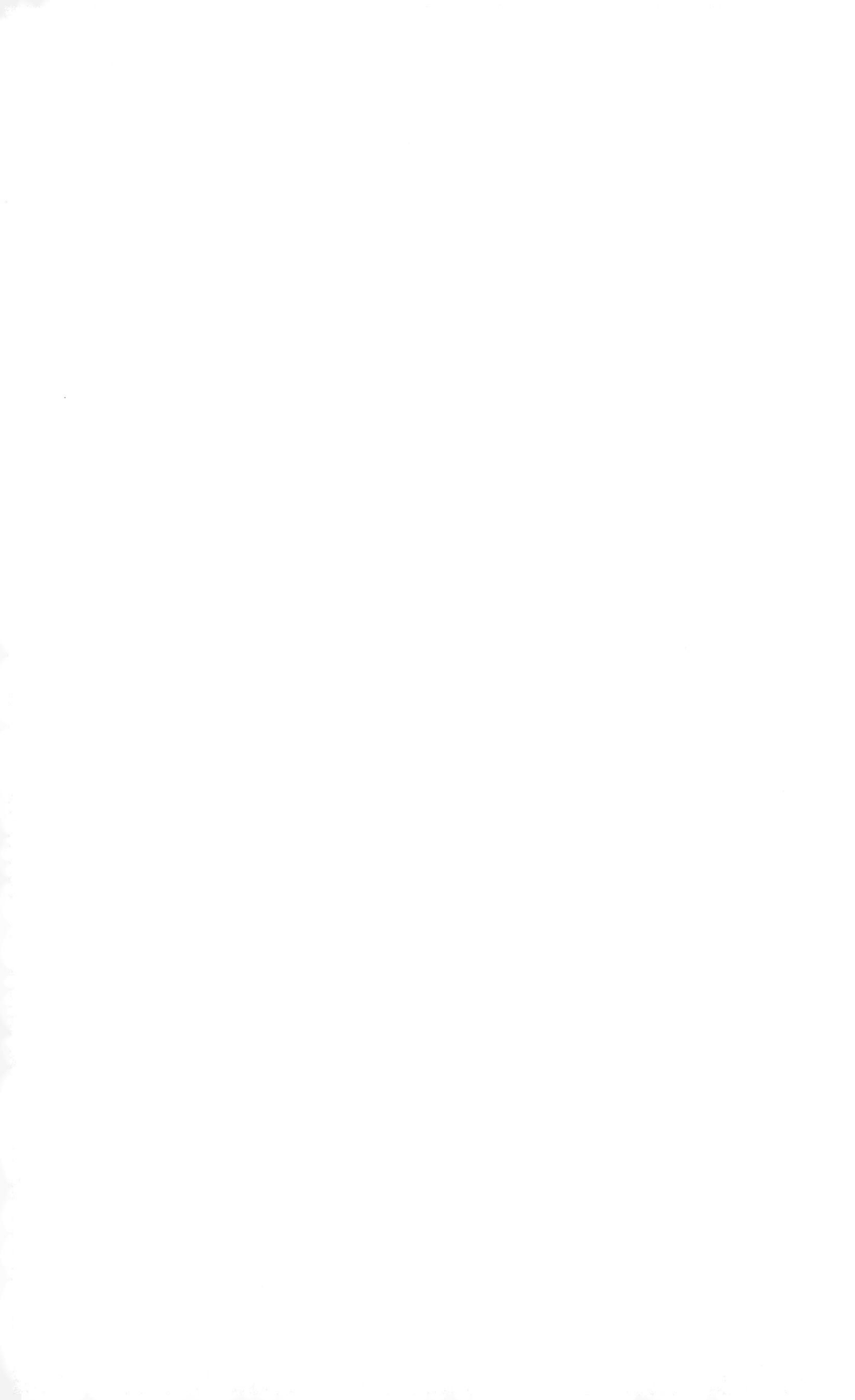

www.ingramcontent.com/pod-product-compliance
Lightning Source LLC
Chambersburg PA
CBHW051422280526
45785CB00003B/1117